Endorsements For *Shuffle: A Way Forward, Whatever the Challenge*

Windy has given us a heartwarming and inspirational look into his personal journey with Parkinson's disease. He shares with us a light-hearted yet powerful story of faith, hope and love. He tells us how his faith in God, his hope for the future and the love for his family have played an important role in managing the impact Parkinson's disease has had on his life. Through this book, Windy has given people with and without Parkinson's disease a special gift—a gift of inspiration for the future.

Marie Jaffe
Executive Director
Parkinson Association of the Carolinas
parkinsonassociation.org

I first read *Shuffle: A Way Forward, Whatever the Challenge* with the thought that it might help me understand the human condition when it is afflicted with Parkinson's disease. Instead, I laughed, I cried, and I came away encouraged and filled with hope. Windy uses his unique ability to relate to his reader the same way he relates to people in face-to-face relationships—with love and respect. This is a book that doesn't preach at you, it draws you in with biblical wisdom and, in the end, you forget it is about a man with Parkinson's. It is about you and me and where we find strength when faced with adversity. Throughout the book there is a central theme that God is in control. There is hope.

Dr. Joe Siragusa
Executive Director
North Carolina Chiroprac

Shuffle

A Way Forward,
Whatever the Challenge

Wendall Woodall

Highway 51 Publishing, LLC
Charlotte, North Carolina
HWY51.com

Published by Highway 51 Publishing, LLC
Charlotte, North Carolina
HWY51.com

ISBN: 0996057005
ISBN-13: 978-0-9960570-0-4

Library of Congress Control Number: 2014905697

The information included in this book is not intended nor implied to be a substitute for professional medical advice.

Front and back cover design: Steven Mast, Glyph Design Group, glyphdesigngroup.com

To all my fellow PWP:
Let's hope together.

CONTENTS

PREFACE

Of the 150 psalms included in the Hebrew Bible, the authorship of one of those ancient poems, Psalm 90, is traditionally attributed to the Jewish hero Moses. Yes, the same Moses who allegedly parted the Red Sea and bore an uncanny resemblance to Charlton Heston.

"Teach us to number our days, that we may gain a heart of wisdom," Moses wrote in Psalm 90:12. My simple take on the meaning? When you realize every day is a gift, you tend to focus on the things that really matter. You don't want to waste a single day. You make a serious attempt to use every second you've been given wisely.

Inspired by the psalmist's words, several years ago I began to keep track of the days I've been alive on the planet. It's an unusual practice, I'll admit, but the potential benefit was compelling. I could become a wiser human being in the process.

I was 17,985 days old when I was diagnosed with Parkinson's disease. As I pen these words, I am slowly inching toward 19,000. My sweet wife, who is quite the flatterer, says I don't look a day over 16,000. Anyway, let's just call it a thousand days of living with my new reality.

The day I heard the diagnosis for the first time, I was actually relieved. Finally, there was a name for these strange symptoms I was experiencing, symptoms I would later discover were textbook signs of this not-so-rare neurological disorder. The gravity of it all did not sink in until weeks later: I had a disease for which there was no cure. "Chronic," my neurologist had said. "And progressive." He can be such a killjoy at times, but I still like him.

Yet, I have made a decision since those early days and weeks of discovering the truth. I can face the future with sadness, despair, and a crippling sense of hopelessness, or I can choose to see each day as a gift that I dare not squander nor take for granted. My doctor explained that while Parkinson's is a disease of inconvenience, it will not necessarily shorten my life. I could easily live to be 29,220 or maybe even the ripe old age of 32,872! That would be a whole lot of days to use wisely, to make the most of, to see as gift-wrapped opportunities to spend the best way I know how ... which is why I have written this book. I want to share the emotions and thoughts that have filled my first 1,000 days— the mere beginning of my path, I know—but also I hope to plot a course for my own heart and mind to follow from the very start. I welcome you along for the ride. I believe it was Confucius who said, "A journey of a thousand miles begins with a single shuffle." Well, at least that's what he would have said if he'd had Parkinson's, like me.

Wendall "Windy" Woodall
Charlotte, North Carolina

HISTORY

All the days ordained for me were written in your book before one of them came to be. —Psalm 139:16

The first symptom I noticed was a shuffling gait that seemed to appear much too soon for a person of my age. I say that about all my abnormalities—the bad knees, the weakening eyesight, the hairy ears, the balding head, and so forth. One of my daughters happened to be home from college and watched me walk across the room carrying a glass and plate to the kitchen.

"Dad, why in the world are you walking like an old man?" she asked.

Maybe it was the fresh set of eyes after being away at school for a while that enabled her to see the change, but my wife, Cheryl, immediately agreed.

"I've been noticing that, too, especially at night when he gets up to go to the bathroom." OK, I didn't list *all* my abnormalities earlier. That particular nocturnal habit started way too soon for me, too, though. The fact is, they were both seeing something that I had been aware of for several months.

I'm not sure how else to explain it, other than that I started finding it difficult to lift my feet when I walked. It

3

wasn't painful, just an annoying mystery. If I concentrated hard enough, I could take long strides as well as the next guy, but when I was tired or just not paying attention, I would quickly slip back into the weary tread of an elderly person. If you're old enough to remember, imagine Tim Conway's white-haired, old man character on *The Carol Burnett Show*.

The slow gait was especially noticeable when I walked the dog every morning, part of my daily routine. The circular route that I followed each day was exactly one mile, a distance I usually covered in fifteen minutes or so. But after a while, the time gradually increased to twenty minutes and then progressively longer as the days went on. By the time my daughter made her observation, it was not uncommon for me to clock in at close to thirty minutes for the same one-mile stretch of sidewalk. That's not exercise, it's a tortoise race. I knew something was wrong.

The medical term for what I was dealing with is *bradykinesia*, although I didn't know the fancy title yet. The word literally means "slow motion" or "slowness of movement." If I had known, I could have volunteered as the poster boy for that particular symptom. Bradykinesia is considered one of the four main indicators of the onset or presence of Parkinson's. The other three are rigidity, tremors and postural instability.

Most doctors would probably say that a single symptom is not enough evidence to cause concern. If two of the four are present, however, you should probably schedule an appointment to check everything out. If three or four are observed, you should go ahead and sign up for the newsletter.

In my case, the measurable decrease in speed was pronounced enough for me to mention it to my general practitioner at my next physical. That one comment—spoken almost nonchalantly as I sat in my backless gown waiting for the OK to get dressed again and get out of there—started me down a road of discovery that would ultimately lead me to the truth. I didn't get there right away, though. It would take a while.

The next step, my family doctor advised, was to see a neurologist. I was nervous, without a doubt, and the nervousness only increased when the new doctor walked in the room looking like he was barely out of high school. I was a high school teacher at the time, and he could easily have passed for one of my students. My confidence in his abilities was not boosted, either, when he began to perform the so-called assessments.

I was expecting highly advanced neurological testing. What I was asked to do instead seemed almost ridiculous, things like touching each of my fingers with the opposing thumb as rapidly as possible; tapping my knee repeatedly with the little rubber reflex hammer; walking on just my tiptoes across the examination room and then returning using only my heels.

The grand finale felt like the silliest request of all: I was asked to stroll down the hallway outside the examination room for about ten yards and then walk back. But as I mentioned earlier, I tended to shuffle along only when I was fatigued or not fully concentrating. If I gave the mechanics of my stride my undivided attention, I could walk like the rest of the human race, at least for twenty yards. And because the neurologist, my wife, and a nurse or two were all watching me walk, I called forth my best effort. I wasn't going to fake shuffle.

Evidently, I passed all the tests with flying colors, because when we sat down together a few minutes later, the doctor asked me: "Now, why were you referred to me? Because, from what I have observed today, there's nothing wrong with you. It might just be psychosomatic."

Cheryl quietly touched my knee in a loving attempt to head off a scene. I think with that one little squeeze, she was trying to remind me that I was also a pastor in the community and that everyone in the doctor's office that day probably knew that, and, therefore, I should act accordingly.

Now, just for the record, I had lovingly done the same thing for her when she was in labor with our third daughter and using a less than ideal vocabulary. I am still healing from the emotional scars of my failed endeavor. Who knew my darling wife had such a temper? I'm hoping she won't read this aside and reopen old wounds. Mine, that is. But I digress. Back to the story.

Being the saintly man that I am, I calmly described for this Doogie-Howser-wannabe the slow, trudging steps that had become part of my everyday routine.

"Well, we'll at least do an MRI so that we can rule out some things," he squeaked in his prepubescent voice as he exited the room. "I'm not really expecting to find anything, though."

Luckily, the door closed before my non-pastoral response was uttered. I'm totally over the whole ordeal now, as you can probably tell. The MRI was promptly scheduled and, as predicted, revealed nothing physical that would explain the bradykinesia. In other words, there was no obvious brain tumor on the pictures, nor could the radiologists see any of the bright, white scar tissue that would have been evident if I had suffered a stroke.

To his credit, the neurologist was systematically eliminating possibilities, which I know proved helpful in the long run, but it certainly was not the conclusive answer that I craved then. He could tell me what I didn't have, but what was my problem, then? Could it be that it *was* all just in my head?

In a manner of speaking, that was exactly what it was.

Later in the process, I discovered that there are no real screening tests for Parkinson's disease. There's not a single examination a doctor can give a patient that immediately diagnoses the disease. All the finger-drumming, knee-tapping, tiptoeing-through-the-tulips exercises that I went through that first day were legitimate methods for trying to determine if there was some kind of disconnect between the brain and the body. The problem with that kind of testing, however, was that in the beginning most of my symptoms were extremely intermittent. I either had simply enjoyed a good day on the morning of my visit to the neurologist, or the increased scrutiny merely enabled me to fully concentrate on the tasks and ace them all, at least neurologically speaking.

For whatever reason, I did look symptom free that day. When I look back, I liken the whole encounter to that of a person taking his or her automobile to the mechanic because of a recurring noise coming from under the hood, only to have the vehicle run smoothly and silently on the day of the visit.

What changed everything was such a small detail that it might easily have been overlooked. If you will recall, there are four major indicators for Parkinson's. If there's just one in evidence, it's probably not a big deal, but two or more could indicate a problem. My last phone call with the young neurologist was conciliatory on his part and enlightening for me.

"I'm going to take your word on the shuffling gait," he said. "But there was another symptom that I noticed that day, and, taken together, they might be significant. Your arms didn't swing when you walked down the hallway and back, so I think I'm going to refer you to a movement disorder specialist."

As with the bradykinesia before, I didn't know the proper medical term, but what the doctor had observed in my stroll were signs of rigidity, basically a stiffness in the arms, legs, or even trunk of the body. My arms did not swing when I walked. For that seemingly irrelevant detail, I was being bumped up to the next guy. It seemed we were getting somewhere.

I'd never heard of a movement disorder specialist before that day. When I met the one who would eventually become my treating neurologist a few weeks later, I asked him almost immediately about the difference between his practice and that of the first neurologist I had visited. Call me gun shy, I guess. I'll concede that I was coming in a little bit leery this time around.

He politely explained that the study of movement

disorders was just one of many subspecialties in the field of neurology. Simply, he had undergone additional training in this one particular area that enabled him to more successfully identify the presence of a movement disorder and thus be able to more effectively treat the patient. He didn't say this in a cocky way, but I got the feeling he did indeed know what he was talking about. I was willing to give him a chance. Plus, he looked like he was older than one of my high school students, which was important to me at this point in my search for an answer. OK, OK, I'm letting it go.

He did, however, start the session by having me tap my fingers together again the same way I had started the previous consultation, and I had to repeat my hallway-walking performances for a small audience. As before, I refused to fake shuffle, and I found myself swinging my arms intentionally. I wasn't going to make this easy.

But then we sat down and he listened intently to my description of the shuffling feet syndrome. He wanted to know when it had started and with what regularity it occurred. If I remember correctly, he nailed me on the exaggerated arm swinging and wanted to know what happened when I wasn't focusing quite so intensely. Then he asked me about other symptoms that I might have observed over the previous months, symptoms that I would not necessarily have associated with the shuffling but which he was obviously linking together.

We began to talk about how my fingers and toes had started to curl inward at random times throughout the day; my legs sometimes refused to stay still when I tried to sleep at night; I had started showering in the evening because it was taking me much longer to get ready for work in the morning; and most recently I had noticed my handwriting was getting sloppier and smaller when I wrote on the board at school. And on it went.

The doctor nodded his head through all these seemingly trivial-to-me details, but the final one appeared to clinch it for him: I reported that there were moments throughout my day when I felt locked in place and could not move without an intentional, sustained effort.

He looked up from his notes and said: "It's called *freezing.*" Then he added, "You have Parkinson's disease. It's considered young-onset Parkinson's because of your age, but all the things you've described point to that diagnosis."

I know it sounds weird now, but, actually, I was relieved to hear the news. Granted, I didn't know enough about Parkinson's, yet, to be too worried, but I felt that being able to put a name on everything I had observed was a good thing. At least now I knew what I was up against.

My first question was simple: "So, what is Parkinson's exactly?" The only thing I knew about the disease was that some very famous people, such as Michael J. Fox and Muhammad Ali, had been diagnosed with it. But I wanted to know what it meant for me.

The doctor explained, in a nutshell, that having Parkinson's basically meant that the brain stops creating sufficient amounts of the chemical dopamine, despite the fact that it needs dopamine to control things such as the movement and coordination of the body. The progression of the disease is different for every person who has it, but there are certain symptoms very common to anyone who has the disease. I'm sure that this is where I learned about the big four that I mentioned earlier.

"It's not fatal," he offered in closing, "but it is chronic, which means there is no cure. All we can do is treat the symptoms."

Did I say I felt relief at first? That was starting to wane.

My second line of questioning was much more direct: "How sure are you about this? And how could you diagnose this so quickly when the first guy said he saw nothing wrong with me?" I realized that just as I was bothered by the seemingly dismissive response of the first neurologist, the immediate certainty of this new one left me equally troubled. But if he sensed the subtle challenge in my tone, he certainly remained cool under fire with his reply.

"It's probably because I focus on just this one area and little else, and because I see these symptoms every day, and yours are textbook. This is Parkinson's; the earliest stages, mind you, but Parkinson's for sure."

I wasn't ready to let go of the uneasy feeling quite yet, so I pushed a little more: "Isn't there a test that I can take to be absolutely, one hundred percent certain? Something a bit more objective?" It all seemed like too big a deal to base on a few strolls down the hallway and a handful of anecdotal responses to questions about my symptoms.

Again, he remained completely calm and said: "There is a test called the DaTscan that has just recently been approved for use in the U.S. It can help confirm the diagnosis but it's expensive, and we'd have to see if your insurance company would approve it."

Now, we're talking, I thought to myself. We could *prove* if I really had Parkinson's, once-and-for-all.

"So, what would this test increase your certainty level to?" I asked. Inside, I was elated. I could get a definitive answer! But then he hit me with the sobering news.

"I'm 98 percent sure right now. With the DaTscan, we could bump that up to 99 percent certainty. So, it's up to you."

The rest of the appointment was a blur. I know that he talked about the importance of exercise and maybe some physical therapy. We discussed medications with names like "agonists" and "inhibitors" and the current gold standard of treatment, something he called "carbidopa/levodopa." He spoke about the need to maintain a positive attitude and guard against negativity. He emphasized the good news that many people with Parkinson's were living long and productive lives. Parkinson's for them was merely a nuisance, he argued, and what he tried to do for his patients was make an extremely annoying disorder a little less annoying. Much of it would depend on me.

I agreed to call back about the DaTscan, and we set up a date for my follow-up visit. (A few weeks later, I did have the "dopamine transporters" scan done, and it confirmed the diagnosis. I guess I needed that other 1 percent of certainty. The bottom line is that the Parkinson's diagnosis seemed to be a sure thing.)

I left the doctor's office that day, walked to my car and called my wife with the news. She tearfully asked how I felt, and I responded with a few one-word descriptors: relieved, curious, anxious, uncertain. We said a short prayer together, and then agreed that I would call my parents and she would call our three daughters.

She asked if I was going to head home right away, but I said no, because I was already right there at the hospital, so I would make a few of my pastoral visits. Then, I'd meet her at the house when she got off work. You shouldn't be too impressed by my stoic reply, however. I wasn't trying to be noble. The truth is that I had no clue what to do in response to my big news. Comforting and praying for a few sick people seemed like a good idea at the time. Maybe I could get in a couple of prayers for me as well.

~

My lovely wife, Cheryl, and I met in college down in Lakeland, Florida, in the early 1980s. We dated off and on for three years, finally got engaged, and then broke up weeks before the wedding. She decided that she didn't want to be married to a workaholic, no matter how good-looking (or humble) he happened to be.

She went back to Texas to finish school, but, for a myriad of reasons, she was forced to come back to Florida for her last year of undergraduate studies. I was still in town, serving as an associate pastor on the staff of a local church. Her sister, Candy, brought her by my apartment to get some of the things she had left behind but now needed to outfit a dorm room once more.

There was a rather lengthy, awkward moment of staring into one another's eyes when I opened the door that hot,

August afternoon. Long story short: eight months later we were married. I guess the good looks won out. Well, at least they did back then. Now, she says she married for love the first time; the next time she's marrying for money. I think she's just kidding.

Anyway, things moved quickly, and by our third year of marriage, we were the parents of two sweet, gorgeous, and intelligent daughters, Brittany and Lauren. Then, much to their grandparents' dismay, while the two girls were still toddlers, we packed up all our belongings and moved to Central America where we would serve as missionaries for the next twelve years.

While we were living abroad, our third, equally sweet, gorgeous, and intelligent daughter, Sarah, was born. With the five of us, our family was complete. We spent a year in Costa Rica to learn the language, but the rest of that time was spent in the lusciously green and picturesque nation of Honduras where we met some phenomenal people, served alongside many capable men and women, and made a handful of lifelong friends in the process. And now, even though we have been back in the States for about as long as we lived in Honduras, we would all say that we are still at least partly *catracho de corazón*—which translates, "Honduran at heart."

So, what's my reason for the short family bio? Well, for one, I always like to talk about my four girls. Cheryl and I wouldn't trade our family for anything in the world. We did discuss somewhere along the way trying one more time for a boy. Then, we met another missionary family in Honduras who had had the same idea. And while we thought their seven daughters were absolutely darling, we also decided that three was an entirely perfect number for us. Who wants to mess with perfection?

The second reason for the bio is this: as a family we learned some extremely valuable lessons during our time in Central America. Our more than a decade of cross-cultural living taught us a thing or two about how to face circumstances in which everything familiar disappears and you have to adapt to a whole new cultural setting. Most people who have lived in another country for an extended amount of time have learned these lessons. Well, that or they've gone home completely frustrated and discouraged.

Our sending agency had learned that lesson well, so, as part of our preparation to head overseas, we thoroughly studied the concept of cultural adaptation. One key to successfully acclimating oneself to a new culture, the trainers taught us, is to first understand the evolutionary process through which everyone must go. There will be three stages, or phases. The first one is called the *tourist*, or *honeymoon* stage. That's when adrenaline levels are high and everyone is both excited and apprehensive. It's followed by the letdown of the second phase, known as *culture shock*. Excitement is replaced by frustration, and a lot of people never recover from this stage. However, if the person is willing to work through this low point of their cross-cultural experience and begins to do what is necessary to emerge on the other side, he or she might just arrive at the third and final stage: *cultural adaptation*. Briefly, cultural adaptation means that the once-excited-and-then-frustrated individual is gradually able to adjust his or her personal habits, customs, and ways of thinking in such a way that they begin getting comfortable in their new culture. That's what most long-term international workers and expatriates living abroad genuinely desire.

Understanding this process from start to finish was crucial to us during our years in Central America. With Parkinson's, it has proven to be extremely useful once again. The progression was the same; we just switched settings. Let me explain a little further, beginning with the tourist stage.

When we first arrived in Costa Rica and, a year later, in Honduras, we looked and acted like tourists in countries all around the world. We were snapping pictures of everything and everybody, sampling the exotic foods and drinks, learning the rudiments of what appeared to be a fascinating local language, and so on. We were encountering everything for the first time and the differences between our home culture in the U.S. and these two new host cultures were the very things that make the move so enjoyable. Who doesn't love a siesta every afternoon? Who wouldn't be flattered by the overly friendly taxi drivers who almost fought for the right to take us wherever we needed? Who couldn't enjoy the refreshing rains that cooled off the city almost every afternoon? Our "honeymoon" phase lasted for well over a year. It can be a much shorter period of time for some people, depending on their individual temperaments and personalities, but it was exhilarating for us while it lasted.

Our family has gone through a similar tourist stage with this new Parkinson's diagnosis. The analogy isn't perfect because I don't think anyone would ever call the first few weeks or months after receiving such sobering news the "honeymoon" period of their experience. Still, my family and I definitely found ourselves in unknown territory, and we looked every bit the part of tourists, just as we had before, with eyes wide open and mouths agape, seeing and hearing everything for the first time. We were learning the medical jargon, sampling the new medications and treatments, taking mental snapshots of the information from every reliable source we could find. I think I read through at least a dozen books on Parkinson's owned by our local library, and my girls bookmarked at least that many websites in our joint exploration of this new place. Curiosity consumed us, and we couldn't take in the sights and sounds fast enough.

Yet, such high adrenaline levels can only be maintained for a brief time. Eventually, routine slips in, the day-to-day living to survive, and slowly, but surely, you begin to notice that the differences you celebrated when you first arrived now are the sources of your greatest frustrations.

Our family certainly went through those ways of thinking during the time we spent in Central America. The adaptation hit a snag or two—or three or four. That relaxing siesta time? It was great until you realized almost all the local businesses closed for two hours every day and the town came to a virtual standstill. Those friendly taxi drivers? They were fighting over us because they knew they could charge us the higher rates, and we cultural outsiders would be none the wiser. That refreshing rain? The wet season lasted for six solid months and mildewed everything we owned—food, clothing, furniture, books, small children and so on.

Both the big and small frustrations accumulated until we reached a tipping point. Then, it seemed like it all became a source of irritation. The anthropological term for this phenomenon is *culture shock*, and it happens to the best of us. Actually, it happens to almost everybody, no matter how tough they are.

Basically, culture shock can be defined as the feelings of disorientation, disillusionment, and depression that an individual faces when the realization finally hits them that the unfamiliar culture in which they now find themselves is their new home, ready or not. Vacationing travelers usually avoid the negative emotions because they're on the plane heading home long before it sets in. But for those who have to stay, the sense of bewilderment is almost inevitable.

The bottom line is that the newness wears off, and you start waxing nostalgic for the way you did things before. If you're not careful, the frustration rushes in like a flood, overflows its banks, and threatens to sweep you down the river like so much driftwood.

So, what do you do then? A lot of people give up and go home or, if they can't do that, they become embittered and never truly adapt to their new home.

With Parkinson's, the truth we had to face was simple: There was no going back for us. Barring a miracle, that was not an option. We were never going to catch the next plane out and return to the normalcy of a pre-Parkinson's world. We were living in the new normal for us, and we were here to stay.

But as time passed, we slowly slipped into culture shock, or maybe a better phrase would be "diagnosis shock." Whatever you call it, the same waves of disorientation, disillusionment, and depression that all long-term residents of new cultures live through threatened to sweep in on us as well.

Our attempt to find the best course of treatment for everyone who had Parkinson's led us to the disheartening discovery that everyone's path is different. In addition, this new world, with its unique language of medications, therapies, clinical trials, and even hints of surgical implants, was perplexing to us. The frustration within began to grow. How would I ever decide which treatments were right for me? Which ones could I tolerate physically and which ones would I not be able to? Which combinations of all of the above would mask my symptoms the best?

Everyone with Parkinson's disease that we knew was either on different medications altogether or vastly differing dosages of the same medications. How could anybody plot out a course with such variables?

I asked my neurologist that very question, and he confirmed what we feared: "We treat every individual according to his or her unique needs and symptoms. There is no one-size-fits-all approach." It was all overwhelming. The bitterness and frustration were just around the corner. We could feel it.

But we made a decision, both in Costa Rica and Honduras back then and now with Parkinson's. We recognized the low point for what it was: an inevitable reaction and a normal part of transitioning from what we were used to doing and the new way we would now need to do things. And we chose to tough it out and do whatever was necessary to not only survive but to thrive in our new place of residence.

Like it or not, this strange land was our home now, so we might as well start settling in and getting acclimated to where life had brought us. We had done that very thing in Central America. We would do the same with Parkinson's. Both then and now, we realized that whatever changes had to be made would need to take place in us, not in the circumstances themselves. That is cultural adaptation: We adapt to the culture. The culture does not adapt to us. I'd like to think I'm already at this third and final stage. It's certainly where I want to be.

So, what do you do to get there? These next few chapters will tell you. They represent the ways of thinking and living that I believe are part of the "whatever is necessary" to get me to that final phase and keep me there. What I'm hoping is that my own journey will help you get there, too.

I'm writing this book especially for those with Parkinson's—my fellow shufflers, if you will. Yet I realize that these truths may help others who have arrived in their own strange, new lands and have a choice to make. You're welcome to join us. Just remember not to walk so far ahead.

HONESTY

But he said to me, "My grace is sufficient for you, for my power is made perfect in weakness." Therefore I will boast all the more gladly about my weaknesses, so that Christ's power may rest on me.
—2 Corinthians 12:9

Our culture doesn't really celebrate weakness. We'd rather highlight the young, the strong, and the healthy. If that is indeed the checklist for life, I'm probably not going to be picked for the team. I was reminded of that fact not too long ago.

I was asked to be one of the male chaperones for a group of high school seniors who were celebrating their upcoming graduation with a weeklong cruise to the Caribbean. I know, I know. You're probably thinking, "What a great perk for a teacher!" But let me remind you that I would go through many sleepless nights trying to keep up with the students. I would have to bunk in close quarters with at least three of those teenagers, in a room really designed for one. Plus, I would bear the somber responsibility of seeing to their safety and welfare for the duration of the trip, serving as the protector of their very lives, if you will.

OK, you're right. It was a nice perk, and I thoroughly enjoyed myself. But I remember something on that particular cruise that I don't think I will ever forget. The boat that week was filled with seniors of both varieties: the high school and college versions, and the AARP kind. Our rooms were on the bottommost passenger deck of the ship, the "cheap suites" we called them. We had to walk up several flights of stairs just to see the sun again, but the daily ascent was worth it. Once you arrived at the top, the scene was glorious: sparkling pools were surrounded by people laughing, dancing, and eating to their hearts' content, not to mention the stunning ocean views for as far as the eyes could see.

On one particular morning, though, I was lucky enough to catch the elevator on the bottom floor just as several sleepy and slightly hung-over college students were cramming in, beginning their daily migration to the paradise at the top. Most of them didn't change out of their bathing suits the whole week.

The elevator stopped at almost every deck along the way. At one of those stops, a white-haired, elderly couple slowly got in. And when I say slowly, I mean it was like watching a snail crawl. Several times, the elevator doors tried to shut on them as they trudged in, leaning on each other for support, and leisurely pivoted to face the front.

I remember thinking how sweet they looked together and what a treat it must have been for them to travel like this during their retirement years. A couple of decks later, they shuffled out through the open doors, step by agonizing step, and the doors eased together behind them as they cleared the threshold. Then one of the young twenty-somethings said to the rest of her crew: "If we could just kill all the old people now, life would be so much better." Everyone laughed but me.

I know I probably should have said something in defense of the elderly around the world, something noble and inspiring that would have melted every heart and transformed forever their perspective on the generations that went before them. But I was speechless, and I found myself instead trying to stand up straighter and look thinner, nervously glancing around to see if anyone was calculating the ages of the elevator's occupants. They were not, as far as I could tell, but I did keep looking over my shoulder for the rest of the week.

The young lady wasn't serious—at least I hope she wasn't—but what she said was indicative of what we appear to value as a culture. I can't say that I ever gave it much thought before the recent events in my life, though. But now that I am less young, less strong and less healthy, I find myself thinking about it more and more. I also have somewhat of a phobia when it comes to large groups of twenty-somethings in elevators, but I'm working through that.

~

If you'll look back at the opening verse of this chapter, you will see that the Apostle Paul, who wrote a good portion of the New Testament, came to think about things a little differently than we do in our present culture. If you're from a religious background, specifically of the Christian persuasion, what I'd like to do over the next few pages is look at the context of this particular verse in the Bible and perhaps see what God was trying to say through Paul in this letter penned to the Corinthians of ancient Greece. If you're not from a religious background, then you have my permission to either skip ahead or just read along for the fun of it. I believe that there might be something of value in these words, but ultimately you'll have to decide that for yourself. I did mention earlier that I was a pastor, right? This is kind of what I do.

Paul of Tarsus purportedly wrote two letters to the Corinthians in the mid-first century. Actually, scholars believe that he may have written more missives to Corinth, but only two survived and later became part of the Bible. In the twelfth chapter of the second letter, or epistle, he describes a problem in his own life that had changed his way of thinking. He talks about something he calls a "thorn in the flesh" that God had apparently allowed him to have "to keep him from becoming conceited." (We'll return to this significant theme of humility in the next chapter.)

He doesn't say what the thorn was specifically, although he does call it a messenger from Satan sent to torment him. While that description seems to point to something ominous and evil, most commentators on this biblical passage believe that he was referring to a physical ailment, perhaps something to do with his eyes. (Check out Galatians 4:15 to see why.)

Although none of us can be absolutely certain as to what Paul was talking about, it is clear that he longed to be delivered from it. The passage says that he pleaded with the Lord three times to take it away from him, but evidently God chose not to heal him. Instead, he answered Paul's prayers with these words: "My grace is sufficient for you, for my power is made perfect in weakness." Astonishingly, Paul responds: "Therefore I will boast all the more gladly about my weaknesses, so that Christ's power may rest on me."

In our society today, we celebrate, reward, and show off our strengths for all to see, but we tend to hide our weaknesses. To actually boast about our weaknesses seems almost absurd, the reverse of what most human beings would do. But the Bible is full of these counterintuitive, upside-down teachings: The last will be first, and the first will be last. He who wants to be the greatest should be the servant of all. We should love our enemies, do good to those who hate us, and pray for those who persecute us. All of those ideas are almost the complete opposite of what we would naturally do, and this idea in 2 Corinthians seems to be of a similar vein. God's power is made perfect in our weakness.

What's my paraphrase? God has a much greater opportunity to show off his strength through those who will admit that they are weak. I happen to believe that he specializes in doing just that in the lives of people on every corner of the planet. And what's his reason? Because then the weak are unable to brag about having done it themselves. It would have to be God, or some other power outside of and greater than themselves, and everyone would know it. Paul nearly says that very thing in his first letter to Corinth: "God chose the lowly things of this world and the despised things—and the things that are not—to nullify the things that are, so that no one may boast before him. ... Therefore, as it is written: 'Let the one who boasts boast in the Lord'" (1 Corinthians 1:28-31).

God's power is made perfect in our weakness. If you read through the Bible from start to finish, you'll find that it's full of individuals and situations where this truth is played out. I'll pick just one to talk about: a reluctant hero from the Old Testament by the name of Gideon. Just to be clear, he wasn't the founder of the organization that places those hardback Bibles in hotel rooms all over the world, but he was the man after whom they named the organization.

If you're new to the Bible, you may not be familiar with Gideon's story. It's found in the Old Testament book of Judges, and it starts out almost comically. The Israelites are in trouble yet again, and they need a deliverer, a warrior hero. So, the angel of the Lord goes to speak to Gideon.

Where does he find him? Well, he's not out training the troops or sharpening his sword. Instead, the angel finds him trying to thresh out wheat secretly in a winepress so the enemy won't see him. The winepress is probably a hole dug down in the ground, and this brave guy is down inside of the winepress, throwing the wheat up in the air to separate the chaff from the grain. Do you get the picture? I can just see Gideon peeking over the top edge, straining to see if the coast was clear, then throwing up wheat, pausing for a minute to listen for the sound of approaching hoofs, then peeking out again, throwing up some more, all the while hoping against hope that no one would see him. The epitome of a hero, right? Then the angel of the Lord arrives on the scene and greets him, "The Lord is with you, mighty warrior!" (Judges 6:12).

Gideon must have thought to himself: "Are you talking to me?" He doesn't look and sound like a warrior, that's for sure, if you go by his location and his reply, which was somewhat less than inspiring.

"How can I save Israel?" he says. "My clan is the weakest in my tribe, and I am the least in my family" (Judges 6:15). He's not exactly exuding confidence. And then he does the whole fleece test, twice for good measure. You'll have to read the story if you don't know what the heck a fleece has to do with all this, but finally he is convinced that it's God talking to him, so he leads an army of 32,000 men and sets up camp just south of where the enemy forces have gathered.

Then, right before the battle is to begin, God does the strangest thing. In order that no one in Israel can boast that their own strength had saved them, he tells Gideon to dismiss everyone who is trembling with fear because of the upcoming skirmish. Incredibly, Gideon complies with God's request and 22,000 men admit they're scared to death and head for home. If you're a little rusty on the math skills, that would leave just 10,000 remaining troops, less than a third of what he started with. And then, as if taking a cruel joke one step further, God tells Gideon that he still has too many soldiers.

At this point, I would have been thinking maybe it was God who was a little rusty on math. But once again, the obedient Gideon obeys and takes the 10,000 men down to the river and, based on the way they take a drink of water, he sends home another 9,700 men. That left a mere 300 men for Gideon to lead into battle, which might have been enough if they had been Spartans and Gideon was more like King Leonidas. But these were no Spartans. That movie hadn't come out yet.

Yet, the number 300 does seem to satisfy God's wish to whittle down the army to the required "no boasting" level, so all is well. I think I would have told God, "Well, that's just great, God. But if you don't mind, I think I'll head back down to the winepress—and not just to hide. I need a drink." He doesn't say that, but I'm betting he thought it.

I don't want to spoil the rest of the story and give away what happens next, but suffice it to say that with a standing army of 300 men, Gideon totally defeats his enemies who, the narrator of this passage says, were as thick as locusts and whose camels could no more be counted than the sand on the seashore. Now, if that were true, the original 32,000 would have represented a miraculous win as well. Winning with 300 made it even more so.

What does this quaint story from the Bible have to do with having Parkinson's? What am I proposing we take from this ancient text? Namely, that we should not presume that, just because of our weakness, be it Parkinson's or anything else, we are already defeated and we have absolutely no hope going forward. Instead of conceding the battle, we should be more determined than ever to do whatever we feel destined to do with our lives, in spite of our weaknesses and regardless of the obstacles. Why? So that others might see the miracle that is our lives and either point to God, which is the option I'm obviously rooting for, or at the very least be so inspired by our unrelenting determination to never give up, never give in, and never say die, that they continue to successfully fight their own battles. And win.

In order for either one of those two things to happen, however, there is a condition that must be met. We will have to be open and honest about having Parkinson's in the first place.

For most of us that's not a difficult task. The telltale symptoms of the disease with which we struggle give away our secret every day. It's hard to hide the obvious. But I'm suggesting something more intentional: boldly and deliberately stepping forward and admitting that we have a weakness. It's called Parkinson's. Except in this scenario, we're not complaining or using it as an excuse to withdraw from life. We're making it our reason to stay engaged. Like the Apostle Paul, we should do a little boasting about our weaknesses, maybe something like this: "I have Parkinson's, but that's not going to prevent me from doing what I feel like I'm supposed to do with my life. It may slow me down, perhaps considerably so, but I will not quit without even trying. Instead, I'm going to continue to fight against this condition every day of my life, the best I know how."

I'm not talking about denial or some kind of motivational mumbo jumbo, nor am I advocating that we sugarcoat the reality of our unique conditions. In varying degrees, we all have physical and mental limitations that we cannot simply ignore or pretend aren't there. No, I am proposing that in the very face of those irrefutable and often limiting symptoms, we continue to shuffle forward, one day at a time, for as long as we possibly can. And I happen to believe that by doing so, we extend the "for as long as we possibly can" even further in our lives. Remember, I count days. So, I'm all about adding as many more as possible to my total. I'm thinking that most other human beings are as well.

There's one more thing that I'm *not* advocating, by the way. Let's not play the sympathy card at any point, so that people will simply feel sorry for us, although, in full disclosure, I have been known to do so, especially when it's time to do chores around the house. It's to no avail.

"You're just milking it," my wife would say. "If you want to be inspirational, vacuum the house." I'm afraid that the sympathy card is not part of a winning hand at my house. But that's OK. We should not be shooting for sympathy or pity, anyway. I believe the end goal is that we inspire ourselves and others by the way we live.

Recently, I was asked to participate in a panel discussion at a symposium on Parkinson's in Charlotte, North Carolina, my hometown. My movement disorder specialist had suggested that I be one of the five to speak briefly on the theme of "Living Well with Parkinson's Disease." I would represent those diagnosed with the young onset version of the disease. I like it when people refer to me as young. If only those twenty-somethings in the crowded elevator could see me now.

Anyway, our facilitator asked us to speak openly and honestly about the struggles we had dealt with thus far in our lives since the diagnosis. But she also asked us to talk about our successes and our determination to continue to enjoy life to its fullest. In an email just a few days before the symposium, she explained why she was looking forward to our part in the program: "We all know that Parkinson's is a very difficult disease and that there is nothing easy about coping with the changes you encounter. We also know that some people seem to cope far better than others, and all of you have inspired us with your ability to adapt, grow, and enjoy your lives despite the challenges you face on a daily basis."

Sound familiar? But if my intention was to inspire others that weekend, I must admit that I walked away even more inspired by my fellow panelists. On my left sat a devoted husband and long-term caregiver who spoke about how he and his wife with Parkinson's planned trips all over the world, taking in to account such issues as mobility, timing, and the need for rest. This was not just theory for them. He and his wife had just returned from a two-week vacation to Italy a few months earlier.

On my right sat an elegant lady and author who had collaborated with her husband on dozens of children's books and travel guides, both before and after she was diagnosed with Parkinson's. She spoke about how they had learned to work together and the adjustments they had made as her symptoms progressed over the years.

Next to her sat a pastor who had the whole place roaring with laughter as he spoke about the inconvenient moments when his symptoms seemed to manifest and of his determined goal to remain active in both ministry and his lifelong hobby of carpentry.

The final panelist was a strapping man who talked about his continuing duties as a girls' basketball coach, even after being diagnosed. Three months prior to the symposium, he had gone through the deep brain stimulation surgery that many people with Parkinson's choose to have. As he finished speaking, he also encouraged the crowd to take up weight lifting as part of their daily exercise regimen, as he had done. It showed.

I left the place believing I could conquer the world, not because I had been moved by some motivational speaker, but rather because what we heard that day came from real-life people with Parkinson's who were continuing to work and play and dream and laugh and genuinely love life. "I have Parkinson's," they said, "but I refuse to give up. I refuse to stop trying. I refuse to surrender to my symptoms."

I briefly shared my own story that day, about working two part-time jobs as a teacher and a pastor, and then getting diagnosed with the disease. In the beginning, I didn't even slow down. Then, about a year and a half later, I was asked to become the full-time assistant principal at the school where I taught. My symptoms were more noticeable by then. I was unsure about how to respond to the offer. So, on my next visit, I admitted to my neurologist all that I was thinking. He asked me what the dilemma was, and I told him that, since I didn't know what the future held for me because of Parkinson's, I didn't know whether to say yes or no.

I'll never forget how he replied, I told the crowd that day: "Don't make the future the determining factor in your decision. Figure out what you can and cannot do today, look at what the job will require of you, and then make your decision based on the present." So, that's what I have done.

I've had to make some adjustments along the way, I explained: small things such as occasionally sitting instead of standing when I teach, and big things like going to bed a little earlier so that I get closer to eight hours' sleep instead of five. But I'm enjoying what I do, and I love the people I work with and the students who come through my classrooms or my office, all of whom know I have Parkinson's and still see me plodding ahead, regardless.

When I later told a colleague about the symposium and having the opportunity to share a little piece of my story and the message that the organizers hoped to convey, he stopped me and said: "Here's what I believe. You may have Parkinson's, but it doesn't have you. You prove that to us every day."

Now, that's what I'm talking about. I couldn't have said it better myself.

~

The day I was diagnosed with Parkinson's, if you will remember, I spoke with my wife first. That was a no-brainer. I called my parents and then spoke with my three daughters. We talked with teary eyes and cracking voices, but no one lost control. That's just not our family.

From there, the news spread rapidly, and that was OK with us. Many well-meaning friends and family members began to contact us. They wanted to show their support and express their condolences. I was grateful for each one. I really was. As you can probably imagine, in my circles there was a lot of talk about prayer and healing and miracles, all of which I am highly in favor of, just for the record. (*Did you hear that, God?*) I can attest to the fact that I have already greatly surpassed the Apostle's Paul thrice-prayed plea asking for God to take this away from me. If the total number of prayers has anything to do with getting an answer, I'm quite sure I'm in the running.

Yet, as a pastor who has visited the sick and the dying throughout decades of ministry, I have seen both sides of the coin as far as answers are concerned. This person was healed, and that one was not. God seemingly listened to his prayer but not hers. One dear friend got the miracle while another friend was not so blessed. Why the disparity?

The truth is: I have no idea. How's that for a theological answer? Anyone who says they do is deluded or a fraud. Is that too much openness and honesty? I know that my "I have no idea" is a very unsatisfying explanation for anyone struggling through the disparity question. Believe me, I know. But the answers that I've been given over the years are just as unsatisfying.

One person says, "It's because you don't have enough faith." But I think even I could come up with faith the size of a mustard seed. (Google that phrase if you don't understand the reference.) Another says, "It's because you have sin in your life." Guess what? We all do. If perfection is the prerequisite, then none of us should expect an answer to prayer.

I think the reasons are much more complex than the feeble ones we tend to offer. My suspicion is that it has something to do with the tapestry of history that God is putting together and the appointed times in which we were all destined to live.

Perhaps Gandalf the Grey, one of my favorite philosophers, said it best in *The Lord of the Rings*. Frodo lamented that he wished that none of their journey had happened.

Everyone who goes through difficult times feels that way, Gandalf wisely responded. But, he continued, it's not something they can decide. We can only choose what we can do with the time we're given.

It's what the Apostle Paul said in Acts 17:26: "From one man he made all the nations, that they should inhabit the whole earth; and he marked out their appointed times in history and the boundaries of their lands."

It's what King David wrote in Psalm 139:16: "All the days ordained for me were written in your book before one of them came to be." I've come to believe that God is orchestrating the details of my life, "for better, for worse; for richer, for poorer; in sickness and in health." I know which three of those pairs of ideas I would prefer for my life, but that's not for me to decide.

Maybe Jesus said it best: "He causes his sun to rise on the evil and the good, and sends rain on the righteous and the unrighteous" (Matthew 5:45). Life brings us both. My part is to choose how I will respond and live out the time that is given to me.

In my mind, I always come back to Paul and his thorn in the flesh. He asked for healing, but he was only promised grace: The grace to endure it; the grace to complete his mission in spite of it; the grace that was sufficient enough to see him through to the end, without his health restored. I know some of my friends who don't believe in God would say that I'm merely explaining away the unanswered prayers, and, quite frankly, I have to admit that they certainly have grounds to believe that. But for me, it was not that Paul's prayers went unanswered. On the contrary, God does answer—Paul even quotes it—but it just wasn't the answer he had hoped for. He asked for healing, but he was only promised grace. Is the latter not God's answer, as well?

~

"Honesty," Benjamin Franklin allegedly said, "is the best policy." I'm not quite sure of the context of that famous quote, but I have come to believe that it's the only way that I can face life: honest about my diagnosis, honest about my weaknesses, honest about my theology, honest about my future. Does anything else really make sense? Not in my humble opinion.

So how is that honesty policy playing out in my life? I have become an avid reader of everything Parkinson's because I truly want to know the unabashed truth. I talk freely with my family and friends about what I'm going through and what may come next, if they ask. There's nothing worse than unsolicited health updates. I mean, we all know that the greeting, "Hi, how are you?" is merely a rhetorical question, right? The bottom line is: I've been upfront and straightforward for most of my life. Why quit now?

As I was closing this chapter, my neurologist contacted me about the possibility of the deep brain stimulation surgery in the near future. I have to be, well, honest. It feels like it's much too soon for me, that I'm entirely too young to be considering that option already. I'll have to do further research and put my doctor through another intense Q&A session. By the time you read these words, however, I most likely will have already made my decision. My wife wants to know if that will mean that I can be controlled by a remote device. If so, she's looking forward to the mute button, the pause, and maybe the fast-forward. I have a feeling that I'll be doing a lot more vacuuming around the house.

HUMILITY

Therefore, in order to keep me from becoming conceited, I was given a thorn in my flesh. —2 Corinthians 12:7

In the summer of 1990, we packed up our whole family and moved to San José, Costa Rica. Cheryl and I were both still in our twenties, and our first two daughters were three and two. Our mission? To make sure our kids lived as far away from their grandparents as possible.

That's not actually true, but we were certainly accused of it a time or two. The real assignment was to spend three trimesters at a Spanish language school in San José that had a reputation for producing fluent speakers within a year. For my wife, who grew up in places like Miami, Southern California, and the border of Texas and Mexico, it was about fine-tuning her phonetics and adding to her limited vocabulary. For me, it was more about being torn limb-from-limb linguistically speaking, crushing my self-esteem to nothing more than dust, and then rebuilding me from scratch—one agonizing verb conjugation at a time.

I remember the speech the school's director gave on the very first day of classes. With a cheery smile, he said: "Welcome to the Spanish Language Institute. And those will be the last words that we speak to you in English this year."

By noon that same day, we were called down to the nursery area where our oldest daughter, Brittany, kept trying to climb over the fence, crying the whole time, "I don't know what they're saying to me." My wife tried to get Brittany down. I tried to climb over the fence with her.

It was a long year for all of us. Looking back now, I can say that it was one of the most humbling periods of my life. For the next twelve months, we became like elementary school children again: we pronounced our vowels and consonants out loud in class, tried to put embarrassingly simple sentences together on command, took vocabulary tests every day, put signs on everything in the classroom and at home with the appropriate Spanish word for each item, planned for our show-and-tell presentations, and so on. All we seemed to be missing were the smiley face stickers on our papers and coloring pages. I watched many grown men and women break under the stress and strain of that year, and it seemed that the more education they had, the greater their collapse.

Now, don't misunderstand me here. Our teachers were as kind as they could possibly be. The problem was that some of the adults-turned-kids-again just could not handle being corrected day in and day out. They were used to getting things right, being in charge, teaching others how to do things—in short, they were used to being in control. We all felt things spiraling out of control that year.

A young doctor from China was studying at the institute and attempted to encourage us. Spanish would be his seventh language to conquer, he explained, and he assured us that it got much easier on the third or fourth language. We told him he might need a doctor if he continued trying to cheer us up.

It wasn't just in the classroom that we were humbled, either. To help us learn the language more quickly, the agency that sent us used a total-immersion theory. From the moment we got off the plane, we were encouraged to start learning how to survive in the new culture on our own. Familiar faces did pick us up from the airport on the night we arrived, but we had to depend on public transportation that entire year at the institute.

On the very first morning, I bravely decided to go out for food and hopped on an old, dilapidated bus that seemed to be headed in the right direction. I took a seat toward the middle, excited about my first adventure.

Now, if you've never ridden a bus in Latin America, you won't be able to grasp how I spent the next few hours. Without realizing it, I had luckily boarded the inbound bus just as it began its route from the outskirts toward downtown. There were plenty of seats, space, and air to breathe. That scenario was rather short-lived, however.

At the next stop, at least thirty people got on the bus, which put us at what I thought was fairly close to capacity. I even got up to offer my seat to an elderly lady and joined the throngs standing in the aisles. Then, we hit the next stop where maybe five people got off and it seemed like another thirty got on. I could barely see out the windows because of the people, and I was at the dead center of this growing mass. At every stop, it only got worse. The few that got off the bus each time said the appropriate words to squeeze toward the doors. Some yelled out, "*Parada!*" to let the driver know that they needed out at the next stop, but I didn't learn that term until days later. In fact, it suddenly dawned on me that I didn't know any of the correct words or phrases—either to make the bus stop or to get the crowd to let me through—much less how to ask anyone the location of the nearest grocery store.

At long last, a group of hot, sweaty people disembarked and carried me along with them. Truth be told, I think I was the only one sweating. They all immediately scattered in different directions. I was left standing on the corner with a second moment of insightful awareness: I didn't know where I was, and, worse, I didn't know how to tell anyone where I needed to go to get home.

Several hours later, I did arrive back at our rental house,

primarily due to the kindness and broken English of a few Costa Ricans I met along the way. My lovely wife opened the door, saw my disheveled hair and bewildered glaze, and spoke the words she sensed I needed to hear most: "Did you get milk?"

Did I mention it was a humbling year?

That same day, I had another brilliant idea. Thinking it would be best to avoid the bus routes for a while, at least until I knew the city and the language a little better, I borrowed a bicycle from another language school student who lived right down the street. I should have suspected there would be trouble when I pedaled off and he was shaking his head quietly behind me. There were nuances of driving in Latin America that I didn't comprehend just yet. They do have traffic lights, stop signs, and speed limits, and most city roads mark the lanes with bright white and yellow paint—but all of these things are considered suggestions rather than hard and fast laws.

Traffic cops were few and far between, and almost all of them were on foot. They were sure not going to chase down anybody who violated the rules. And another surprise awaited me: drivers love to blow their horns. My Honduran friends would later tell me that if you only had enough money to either fix the brakes or the horn, you always chose the latter.

And, so, I ignorantly pedaled into this chaotic scene and noticed much too late that the volume of traffic was increasing rapidly around me. Then the two-lane road unexpectedly became a four-lane highway—and I use those terms loosely. That's how many lanes were painted on the blacktop, but we easily had six or seven lanes squeezed into that tight space, and nobody was slowing down. Lines were suggestions, remember? And while I had heard horns blaring sporadically around me up until then, I was now in a cacophony of sound that was literally deafening.

I know what you're probably thinking. I'm one of those people who shouldn't be allowed to roam free without supervision anywhere on the planet. I might have come to that conclusion as well, had I had a spare moment, but there was no time. The four lanes became six officially—and closer to eight or nine unofficially—and that's when I saw it: a huge roundabout.

This was a huge, circular intersection, easily six lanes across, fed by four main highways that converged into one giant merry-go-round of merging traffic, complete with a giant statue of an undoubtedly important historical figure sitting on a concrete island right in the center of it all. I should have gotten his name, for he would become my constant companion for the next sixty minutes or so. I'm not exaggerating. I had been following hard on the bumper of a taxi driver who seemed to know where he was going, so when he darted toward the innermost circle of the roundabout, I was on his tail. And then he deserted me, without so much as a beep of the horn in goodbye, shooting between cars to catch his exit about three-fourths of the way around the intersection. I was left behind to look for my own gap in a sea of bumper-to-bumper traffic. It was the scene right out of *National Lampoon's European Vacation* when Chevy Chase gets on the roundabout with his family and circles for the rest of the day and into the night. But at least Chevy had a car.

I can say this about my misfortune that day: I did feel closer to God. And He must have heard my prayers, because about an hour later a break in the traffic opened up that to my eyes was equivalent to the parting of the Red Sea. I raced across all six lanes, screaming at the top of my lungs, while right on my heels vehicles blared their horns.

When I trudged through the door that afternoon, barely safe and sound but alive, I fell exhausted into a fetal position on the couch. My wife came in from the bedroom, where she had been busily unpacking our suitcases and boxes all day, and said, "So, did you get the milk?"

I love that woman, but she was starting to get on my nerves. She did offer to walk the bicycle back to the neighbor's house for me, though, and when she returned, she had a carton of milk in her hands.

"Did you know there's a little convenience store on the block right behind us?" she asked. "They call it a *pulpería*, or something like that. That'll probably come in handy."

I ate my cereal dry that night. It was better than the humble pie.

~

Let's return to 2 Corinthians 12 and Paul's "thorn in the flesh," a physical ailment of some kind that he was suffering from and prayed repeatedly for God to take away from him, but God evidently did not choose to heal him. What has always caught my attention in this passage is the reason that Paul gives for God allowing this to happen to him.

In the verses immediately preceding the text in question, Paul shares with his readers that he had been granted the high honor of being allowed to see "paradise" and to hear what he refers to as "inexpressible things," things he was not permitted to talk about with anyone. For most people, that kind of insider information on God would have made them arrogant and conceited, and I believe that's exactly the point Paul is trying to make in this passage: "Even if I should choose to boast, I would not be a fool, because I would be speaking the truth. But I refrain, so no one will think more of me than is warranted by what I do or say, or because of these surpassingly great revelations. Therefore, in order to keep me from becoming conceited, I was given a thorn in my flesh, a messenger of Satan, to torment me. Three times I pleaded with the Lord to take it away from me. But he said to me, 'My grace is sufficient for you, for my power is made perfect in weakness.' Therefore I will boast all the more gladly about my weaknesses, so that Christ's power may rest on me" (2 Corinthians 12:6-9).

The clear implication is that God had been the one to give him this burden—in order to keep him humble. I find this to be an absolutely intriguing idea, for both theological and personal reasons. Would God do that? Could that be why

God has allowed this infirmity in my life? To keep me from being too proud? To help me be a more humble person?

I've thought about that possibility often. I'm not trying to equate myself to the Apostle Paul in any way, but we all have talents and gifts and resources that might tend to make us a little too cocky, a little too sure of ourselves, a little too self-sufficient. The trouble is that once you realize that pride is a problem, you can't just flip a switch and suddenly you're humble. You can't just say, "I think I'll be more humble today. In fact, I'm going to shoot for being the most humble person on the planet." It obviously doesn't work that way.

Humility is one of those virtues that is easily lost, usually at the first sound of approval or applause. In fact, I would say that most of the time it's going to take an outside agent or set of circumstances to move us toward humility, almost as if we all need our own thorn in the flesh. That's a scary thought, isn't it? But it's often in our pain and suffering that we're paying the most attention.

Atheist-turned-Christian-philosopher C.S. Lewis once wrote in his book *The Problem of Pain* that people can ignore pleasure, but pain demands their attention. He explains further that pleasure is God's whisper, but pain is his shout— his megaphone to an unhearing world.

I can tell you this: he's got my attention.

~

There's one more Costa Rica story that I must include, because it directly ties 2 Corinthians 12 to our year at the Spanish Language Institute. One occasional coping mechanism we employed in San José was conducting church services in English for anyone who wanted to attend. Almost all of us were involved in local, Spanish-speaking churches on the weekends, but we also looked forward to the times when we could sing, talk, and listen to one another in our mother tongue, English. The meetings also afforded us the chance to commiserate about the trials and tribulations of learning this new language. Let's just call those times together what they really were—therapy sessions.

I'll never forget at one particular English service, one of our fellow students opened his Bible to 2 Corinthians 12 and announced that he had figured out what Paul's thorn in the flesh actually was. We were listening.

"It's been staring us in the face all this time," he said. "The key is when he says that he prayed three times for God to take it away from him. He has to be talking about language school—three trimesters' worth. Learning a new language and a new culture had been his thorn in the flesh."

We all cheered and clapped and agreed that it was indeed an insightful look into the true meaning of Paul's malady. It all fit. Language school definitely kept us from becoming conceited, just like the verse said. And at times we all did feel like we were being tormented, especially in phonetics class. And most of us did secretly think on our worst days that the whole idea of learning a new language and adapting to a new culture was straight from the devil himself. It all made perfect sense. And, as you may have noticed, we really did need therapy.

~

Humility is not often considered a desirable attribute in Western civilization. In fact, most people would probably view it as a real hindrance to continued advancement and success. Humility makes us appear weak, and weakness is not a virtue as far as our culture is concerned. Today, it's all about self-confidence, willpower, and a good dose of swagger. But what does it actually mean when we say that someone is humble or has humility?

Etymologically speaking, both words come from the same root *humus*, which is the Latin word for "earth" or "ground." If you like to think in word pictures, here's an image for you. In the 1956 musical film, *The King and I*, the governess Anna is told of the ancient custom that no one's head should be higher than the king's, in order to demonstrate the proper respect for his sovereignty. The king subsequently toys with her, first by sitting, then by lying on his side and finally sprawled out completely on the floor, movements she has to mimic, only slightly lower each time, to show the honor due the king. That is the perfect picture of humility: Someone who sinks to the "ground" in recognition of their more lowly position, rank, or status.

But being humble can also refer to someone who simply has the good sense to not think too highly of themselves, despite perhaps having every reason to do so. They are self-effacing when it comes to their own importance, and they do not consider themselves as better than others. Their humility, I would argue, may stem from the fact that they remain well-grounded and down-to-earth, two ideas that trace back to that root word *humus* once again. We've probably all said about someone, "He's so rich (or talented or famous—you fill in the blank), yet when you really get to know him personally, he's actually very down-to-earth." That's humility.

And that's the kind of humble disposition the Apostle Paul is talking about and demonstrating in 2 Corinthians 12. He certainly had sufficient cause to brag about his inside track to God. There's no doubt he could have made a boatload of money if he had penned a tell-all of the revelations God had given him. He did write about some of those revelations and those writings became part of the New Testament. But he's also clear that he was forbidden to even mention some of the other things he had seen. In other words, he knew things about God that nobody else knew. Let's face it. Some of us would have been letting the whole world know. We would have bought a tour bus and started our own television network.

"Yet, in order to keep me from becoming conceited, I was given a thorn in my flesh," Paul wrote. And that was the problem in a nutshell. Here was a healer who did not receive healing himself. Here was a believer who demonstrated great faith but evidently did not have enough for his own sake. He wrote in one of his letters that everything should be taken to God in prayer, but he had one glaring request that went unanswered. The apostle who famously admonished others to pray without ceasing and to give thanks in all circumstances had one set of circumstances that he could not easily explain. If Paul were prone to brag, this issue would have stopped him in mid-sentence. "If you believe God can heal, why doesn't he heal you?" the crowd would have shouted. So Paul became what I like to call a wounded healer, someone who suffered just like the rest of us but kept on going, kept on praying, and kept on believing. That's my kind of guy.

~

Parkinson's is my thorn in the flesh. If I have ever even thought about saying that I had all life's answers, those days are long gone. If I have ever even toyed with the possibility that I could control the destiny of my own life, that idea has been permanently removed. I would laugh at anyone who said it in front of me now—respectfully—but I would still laugh. I wasn't exactly an arrogant man before all this happened, but I could be prideful and smug when I was feeling full of myself, and, oh, how I loved to be *right*. Even some of that is being chipped away as I face this new life.

Parkinson's has humbled me in ways that I needed to be humbled. *Humble* is also a verb, you see. It means, literally, "to be brought down low" or, as I like to say it, "to be knocked senselessly to the ground for the ten count: jaw broken, nose bleeding, eyes swollen." OK, that may be a bit much, but you get the idea. For me, it's like the parents who have their first child and everything goes smoothly as the child quickly grows up. Then the second one comes along, and they have another episode of problem-free parenting. They start thinking that maybe it's because they're doing everything right and their parenting skills are obviously far beyond the skills of other mere mortals.

"We should write a book," they say, "and share our

secrets with the rest of the world." And then one of two things inevitably will happen. A third child is born, one who has been sent by God to rock their world. The first two were dreams come true. The third one is a nightmare, and the book never sees the light of day, probably because the third kid burned it in the basement with a blowtorch. The other possibility is that the first two become teenagers. Enough said.

~

There's a third word that comes from that same root *humus*, and that's the word *humiliate*. If to humble someone is to bring them down a notch or two, quietly but efficiently, then to humiliate someone is do it and then post the video on YouTube for the whole world to see, maybe even pulling their pants down for good measure. Parkinson's not only humbles you; it has the real potential to humiliate you, too. I'm in the early stages, so my journey has barely begun, but already I have been embarrassed by this disease. Let me explain.

Parkinson's has both motor and non-motor symptoms. The former have to do with movement, coordination, and mobility. I'll get back to those in a moment. The latter are less visible and include having trouble sleeping, dizziness due to a drop in blood pressure, loss of your sense of smell, loss of sexual drive, mood disorders such as anxiety or depression, and so on. This list is not exhaustive, but you get the picture—not a picnic, for sure. But the thing about the non-motor symptoms is that they are not always noticed by others and won't necessarily draw attention to your condition, unless you're asked to stop and smell the roses and suddenly everyone gasps, "Horrors, he can't smell!" There are worse things.

However, Parkinson's is better known for visible motor symptoms. In fact, everyone will notice these. Long before I was diagnosed, I watched the opening ceremony of the 1996

Olympic Games, held in Atlanta. At the last minute,
Muhammad Ali stepped out to light the torch that would
mark the commencement of the games. The crowd roared
when it saw the former Olympian and gold medalist after
what seemed like years of seclusion. Then we all understood
why he had stepped away from the limelight. It was an
inspiring moment in Olympic history but deeply saddening at
the same time to see this former professional boxer, once
dubbed "The Greatest," as he displayed one of the most
infamous motor symptoms, tremor at rest. The whole world
watched as Ali held the torch with his right hand and his left
hand shook uncontrollably. Occasionally, he reached over
and used his left hand, too, and the tremor would stop. That's
why it's called "tremor at rest." If the hand is engaged in
some kind of activity, it usually ceases to shake, but if not,
then the symptom is quite obvious and humiliating. But who
was going to tell Muhammad Ali that the shaking thing must
have been embarrassing for him? I would have been afraid
that he would decide to engage that left hand upside my head.

Previously, I described my most prevalent symptoms:
bradykinesia, the slow shuffling gait, and rigidity, the stiffness
of movement usually observed in the upper body for me.
When my meds are doing what they're supposed to do and
I'm exercising and getting the rest that I need, these
symptoms are sometimes barely noticeable. But if I've been
negligent or I'm at the end of a pill cycle, or, as I have noticed
recently, the medications are simply wearing off sooner and
sooner, then I can be a shuffling fool with almost no
movement of my torso or arms. I look like a bad impression
of a stiff-walking robot as I cross the room in front of my
students, stroll down the aisle of a grocery store, or walk to
the front of a stage to speak in public. "And please welcome
our guest as he comes to share from his heart today. OK, he's
still coming. Almost here. You're so close! You know, folks, I
think we have time for one more round of applause as he
comes. Maybe two." I would most likely engage my hand
upside the head of that smart-aleck, too. If I could catch him,

that is. I've never had anyone do that, but I have felt all eyes in the room on me as I walked to the beat of my own slow drummer. It is a bit humiliating.

There are other motor symptoms that may or may not be part of my future. Every person with Parkinson's has a unique path that he or she must travel. However, some very common symptoms would include *postural instability*, which is an imbalance issue when standing upright; *micrographia*, which is the development of gradually smaller and smaller handwriting; *akinesia*, also known as freezing, where your feet feel stuck to the floor and it requires a conscious effort to begin moving again; and *dysarthria*, which is the slurred and/or mumbled speech and softness of voice that many patients exhibit. There are others as well, but I've mentioned these four because I have experienced each of them in varying degrees over the last two years. Does that mean they will all become full-blown symptoms in my life? No one knows, but I feel some more loss of dignity coming on. I haven't even mentioned *dyskinesia* yet, those jerky, repetitive movements that are a side effect of the medications that I take, not of the condition itself. Isn't that a catch-22? I can either refuse to take the meds and thus suffer from the disease-related manifestations, or I can reduce the occurrence of those manifestations in my life by taking the meds and thereby create a whole new one. What to do? What to do?

~

As I see it, I only have one of two choices when it comes to the humiliation factor. I can be so overwhelmed by the embarrassment that I crawl back into my bed and hide under the covers, avoiding all human contact. Or I can accept the fact that there will be awkward moments ahead and learn to live with them.

The other day I was preparing to speak in front of the school faculty and I purposely got there early so that I could set up my own podium. It's a small school, and we all know each other fairly well. Everyone is aware that I have Parkinson's, but I still wanted to put a table in front of my chair and sit down to speak so I could hide the tremor that plagues my legs at times. I may be a stiff robot in my upper body, but sometimes I'm all Elvis Presley in the lower half. A dear friend overheard my reasoning, came over to put a hand on my shoulder, and said, "Just embrace it. It is what it is. Nothing is going to change the fact that we know and love you."

Those words of encouragement were kind of humbling, too. Yet, it was the type of humbling that I didn't seem to mind so much. I know there are times I tend to get overly concerned about what other people think or what they might say behind my back. I don't want pity, and I don't want others to feel sorry for me. That's not my style. But I do like this idea of being known completely and loved unconditionally. I happen to believe that's what God is all about, but I also consider it a marvelous thing when it takes place between humans as well.

HELP

Serve one another humbly in love. —Galatians 5:13

I attended my first support group meeting for Parkinson's patients and care partners in the January following my August diagnosis. That's significant in that it took me that long to admit that I might not be able to handle this on my own and that I could probably benefit from the perspective of others who were facing the same uncertain future. I discovered a website for the Parkinson Association of the Carolinas, which published a list of all the groups that met in and around the Charlotte area. Until then, I don't think I was ready to make such a visit. Maybe I was still in shock from the news or even in denial somewhat. But five months in, I finally decided it was time to explore the network of people with Parkinson's in my area, the PWPs they're called. My wife said five months is actually a fairly quick decision for a man. She seemed very proud.

I was no stranger to support groups. I had facilitated one at our church for people with addictions of various sorts. It was called Celebrate Recovery, and it was almost identical to an AA meeting but with a decidedly Christian emphasis. Or, as I like to say, it was an AA meeting returning to its roots. In addition, I helped a husband and wife start a support group called DivorceCare. You can guess what that one was all about. My point is that I already recognized the value of people getting together who were going through similar circumstances. The meetings I oversaw provided people the opportunity to hear one another's stories and in the process draw support from each other. Many lasting friendships were forged during those weekly get-togethers, some of which extended well beyond the walls of our meeting rooms.

Thus, it was not a real big step for me to seek out a group of people who had been affected by Parkinson's for the sake of mutual support and encouragement. The biggest challenge I faced was to find a group of people somewhat close to my own age. Having young onset Parkinson's is its own curse, I guess. Statistically, most people with Parkinson's are age sixty and above. So, where's a young fifty-year-old to go?

A good friend of mine was also diagnosed with young onset Parkinson's a few years before I was. The weird thing is that he's a teacher at my school. As far as we can tell, it's purely a coincidence. We asked the science teachers to check the water supply for good measure, but the results were inconclusive. Anyway, we both were invited to a conference on Parkinson's held at a nearby hospital and decided to check it out.

We arrived a little early, selected a few appetizers from the snack table, and sat down to await the start of the meeting. I noticed first thing that most of the people coming in had ten or twenty years on us, easily. A handful were even older. I couldn't tell what Vince was thinking, but my mind immediately went to: "The two of us stick out like sore thumbs. We don't belong here."

Apparently, I was looking at the glass half empty because at that exact moment Vince leaned over and whispered, "It looks like we're the young studs of Parkinson's disease." I'm not really sure about that stud part, but I do like hanging around Vince. I always walk away feeling better about myself, with a little swagger in my shuffle, as it were.

So, getting back to that brisk afternoon in January, there I was, checking out one of the support groups on my list. I walked shyly into the room full of about a dozen strangers, shook hands all around and sat down at one of the tables that were arranged to form a U-shape in the center of the room. Once again I felt somewhat out of place because of my age, but I was curious. This particular group met at the local YMCA, which also provided a program called RENEW (Research and Education in Neuro-wellness), specifically designed for those with Parkinson's. The idea was that a person could go straight from the group meeting to the physical therapy program led by the Y's trained professionals. It was a convenient, win-win setup for everyone. It was also an easy choice for me. Many of the other groups that met in my area held their monthly meetings in assisted living homes, and most of the attendees were residents in those facilities. I think I would have felt even more like an outsider had I visited those groups. So, I opted for the Y, and it turned out to be a great choice.

To this day, I consider the timing of my visit providential. Here's the reason I even entertain that thought: On the evening of my first visit to a support group that I had picked out of a long list from the Internet, they had invited a guest speaker. Her name was Marie, and she was the newly appointed executive director of the Parkinson Association of the Carolinas, the same organization whose website had published the list! She even opened the meeting that night by saying that she seldom got to visit any of the local groups but had decided to make an extra effort to be at our meeting on that particular night.

I was all ears.

Marie explained that their goal was to help people with Parkinson's maintain their independence, stay active in their communities, and enjoy the highest possible quality of life. She had my attention from the very start. I e-mailed her the next day and asked if she needed volunteers to assist in the office or anywhere else. She responded with an enthusiastic yes, and a beneficial relationship of involvement and service began for me. I was thrilled. My network of Parkinson's people had started and would continue to grow.

~

In Galatians 5:13-14, the Apostle Paul wrote: "You, my brothers and sisters, were called to be free. But do not use your freedom to indulge the flesh; rather, serve one another humbly in love. For the entire law is fulfilled in keeping this one command: 'Love your neighbor as yourself.'" Yes, I know I'm quoting Paul again, but that's mainly because he wrote a big chunk of the New Testament and is, therefore, kind of hard to ignore. Galatians is most likely one of the first epistles he wrote. His main purpose? To settle an argument.

The first Christians were Jewish followers of Jesus who came to believe that he was the prophesied Messiah to come. And as they began to spread the news, many non-Jewish (a.k.a. Gentiles) began to believe as well. The problem arose when some of the Jewish followers began to argue that the non-Jewish followers had to first "become" Jews before they could be Christians. Among other things, that meant getting circumcised. But Paul argued that all the Gentiles had to do was to put their faith, or trust, in Jesus—nothing more, nothing less. No circumcision was required, he said, and he had a rather blunt suggestion for the ones who came up with that idea. (See Galatians 5:12 for a verse I bet you didn't know was in the Bible.) His bottom line was that all believers, both Jews and Gentiles, became Christians by grace through faith. The circumcision group was furious. The non-Jews were ecstatic. No law! No rules!

It's at this point in the argument, however, that Paul writes: "But do not use your freedom to indulge the flesh; rather, serve one another humbly in love. For the entire law is fulfilled in keeping this one command: 'Love your neighbor as yourself.'" Here's my paraphrase of the whole passage:

"It's true that you're free from all that legalistic stuff, but don't use your freedom to please yourselves. Instead, use it to lovingly serve one another, because all that legalistic stuff can be summed up in one command: love your neighbor as much as you love yourself."

How do you love your neighbor? By humbly serving them. And how will they show their love back to you? By humbly serving you in return. It's a radical idea, I know, but if it were genuinely practiced, it would change literally every relationship in our lives. Jesus once said that the distinguishing mark of his followers would be the way they loved one another. Paul is here linking the two ideas together: the best expression of that distinctive love that Jesus talked about is mutual service.

The Apostle Peter agreed. In his first letter, chapter 4, he writes: "Above all, love each other deeply, because love covers over a multitude of sins. ... Each of you should use whatever gift you have received to serve others, as faithful stewards of God's grace in its various forms. ... If anyone serves, they should do so with the strength God provides, so that in all things God may be praised through Jesus Christ" (1 Peter 4: 8, 10, 11). Both Peter and Paul taught this same idea: you love by serving.

Yet, one thing I've learned is that, while we may all agree with that idea in theory and as a matter of principle, it's the "doing" part that gets difficult. It doesn't come naturally to us. It goes against our human nature. All of us tend to watch out for ourselves first and think of others later—after we've had our turn.

At the school where I work, I've never seen a student running as fast as he can for the swings on the playground, shouting at the top of his lungs, "I'll go last! I'll go last! I'll go last!" It just doesn't happen.

It's like the two brothers fighting over who gets to eat the first pancakes at breakfast one morning. The mother sees a teaching moment and says, "You know, if Jesus were here, he would probably say, 'I'm going to let my brother have the first pancake.'"

So, the oldest thinks about that for a minute, then turns to his younger brother with a smile and whispers, "OK, *you* be Jesus." We all like to be served much more than we like to serve.

But then Jesus comes along teaching a seemingly upside-down truth: "Whoever wants to become great among you must be your servant and whoever wants to be first must be slave of all. For even the Son of Man did not come to be served, but to serve and to give his life as a ransom for many" (Mark 10:43-45). In Luke 22:26-27, he says it this way: "The greatest among you should be like the youngest, and the one who rules like the one who serves. ... I am among you as one who serves." Did you catch that? Jesus says that even he came to serve.

In no place in the Bible is that more dramatically demonstrated than in John 13. The passage reads: "Jesus knew that the Father had put all things under his power, and that he had come from God and was returning to God, so he got up from the meal, took off his outer clothing, and wrapped a towel around his waist. After that, he poured water into a basin and began to wash his disciples' feet, drying them with the towel that was wrapped around him. ... When he had finished washing their feet, he put on his clothes and returned to his place. 'Do you understand what I have done for you?' he asked them. 'You call me "Teacher" and "Lord," and rightly so, for that is what I am. Now that I, your Lord and Teacher, have washed your feet, you also should wash one another's feet. I have set you an example that you should do as I have done for you. ... Now that you know these things, you will be blessed if you do them'" (John 13:1-5, 12-15, 17).

This is an absolutely amazing passage if you think about what's going on here. This is the night before Jesus would be crucified. I think I would have been soaking up the sympathy and milking the pity factor for all it was worth. But Jesus, God in the flesh, instead chooses to wash the dusty, stinking feet of his disciples. I'm floored every time I think about it. What's his point? He states it quite clearly: "I have set you an example that you should do as I have done for you." If you're familiar with their story, you know that these are the same guys who continually argued about who was the greatest among them. Nobody wanted to be second, much less last. So, I can just see the scene when Jesus made that last comment: "Do as I have done." The disciples probably looked at one another and whispered: "OK, you be Jesus!"

~

What does all that have to do with Parkinson's? Just this: It's going to take these two ideas of mutual love and mutual service to get all of us through this mess. None of us, patients or care partners, will be able to do it alone. We're going to need each other, whether we're comfortable with that idea or not.

A friend's social media post the other day jumped off the screen at me: "I agree that no man is an island, but I think I am a peninsula." I totally get that. I'm not so arrogant as to think I could do all of life, much less Parkinson's, without help. And yet at the same time I have never liked the idea of having to depend on someone else for anything. It's a pride issue, I know, but I no longer have the luxury of that kind of thinking. I'm going to need a whole network of supporters, both professional and personal. The sooner I understand that, the better.

~

The first people we need in place are the members of our healthcare team. That would include our primary care doctor and our treating neurologist. In my case, the neurologist also happens to be a movement disorder specialist, with additional training and practice in treating those with Parkinson's. That's a clincher for me. I would also say that the neurologist should be someone with whom you feel totally comfortable and in whom you have complete confidence. I admittedly began with a good dose of skepticism but the compassionate and patient bedside manner of my neurologist slowly but surely won me over. Ditto for his entire staff, past and present. (Here's to you, Sarah and Tangela.) I actually look forward to our visits together. I always come loaded with a question or two about what I'm seeing or how the meds are working or what's next, and he always methodically works through the answers with me, doing more listening than talking. I try not to take advantage of his busy schedule or monopolize his time. There are other patients, or so I've heard. But he never seems to be in a hurry, and I always get the sense that he's willing to stay for as long as necessary. Ideally, I think that's how it should be between every doctor and patient.

We've reached an almost jovial relationship. I told him early on that one of the main reasons I trusted him is that when he talks, he looks just like my brother-in-law. My wife confirmed it when she came on one of my visits. "Oh, yeah, handsome as all get out." He was extra patient that day.

On another recent visit, he was typing out his instructions for me as we finished up our conversation. As he punched the last key, he looked up and asked me if there was anything else he could do for me. I immediately quipped, "Yeah, I'd like you to come up with a cure for Parkinson's by next Christmas."

Without missing a beat, he responded, "You'll be the first person I call, I promise." We both laughed as he stood to leave, but then he turned back at the door and added, "No, actually you would probably be the second person. I think I'd get in touch with my financial adviser first." I like an honest man.

There are other healthcare professionals that need to be included, either from the start or as the disease progresses: a trusted pharmacist, perhaps a certified counselor or two, and then various therapists as the needs arise—occupational, speech, physical, and so forth.

I did several months of exercises with a physical therapist right after the diagnosis, until the health insurance company said I had reached my limit. The therapy emphasized exaggerated movements of the arms, legs, and body. The tendency of the dopamine-deprived brain, evidently, is toward smallness—smallness of step, smallness of range of motion, smallness or quietness of voice, and so forth. Thus, to combat this smallness factor, the physical and speech therapy often recommended is referred to as BIG™ and LOUD™, respectively. (See lsvtglobal.com for more information.) As my physical therapist explained, a person with Parkinson's who learns to walk with deliberately long strides, swinging their arms in wide arcs on both sides, is actually just beginning to look like any other person walking down the street. The intentionality of the exaggerated movements only gets me back to normal. I can assure you, however, that it certainly felt abnormal to move around that way, but by this time in my Parkinson's journey, I was used to performance walking on command. I've started thinking about a second career as a runway model.

~

Beyond the medical support team, there also needs to be a personal support team. These individuals are often called *care partners*, in order to distinguish them from the professional caregivers. They are the loved ones who come alongside to help the person with Parkinson's. In the majority of the cases, it's the spouse who is thrust into that role, and I use that word *thrust* deliberately. It means to be pushed or forced into the position. Others may assist—children, grandchildren, close friends, and maybe even parents or siblings, in the case of young onset Parkinson's—but let's face it: it's the spouse who will bear the brunt of the load, ready or not.

I often think about that fact, and sometimes I wrestle with an enormous amount of guilt. You're probably thinking

I shouldn't feel guilty about something that is beyond my control, to which I would lovingly reply, "Mind your own guiltiness." No, the truth is that I know all that, and as a pastor I've even said similar words to others, but I still feel the twinges to some degree almost every day. The bottom line is that I wish I could spare my wife and daughters from all that may possibly come, from the burden that I may one day be to them. But I know I cannot, and so the guilt remains.

Most of that line of thinking comes from the way I was raised and the era in which I grew up. As children we were taught—at school, church, and home—to take responsibility for ourselves, to work hard to provide enough for our own family, and to never ask someone else to do what we should be doing for ourselves. Back then we often heard it preached, "God helps those who help themselves," and we bought into that idea. I'd like to note, however, that this adage is not found in the Bible. I think Benjamin Franklin actually said it, and, while it certainly sounds reasonable, I now know it's not exactly biblical. A more biblical idea would be that God helps those who cannot help themselves—the powerless, the defenseless, the helpless. Even so, how do you remove eighteen plus years of believing the opposite? When I fast-forward to the present and my new existence of weakness and vulnerability, I find myself overwhelmed when I consider that one day I may not be able to do everything for myself anymore. I'll have to learn to let others serve me. It's not going to be easy.

~

The reality of my diagnosis on that August afternoon two years ago is this: It wasn't just me on the receiving end. It hit my wife and our three daughters just as hard. However, there's no doubt in my mind that my sweet, compassionate, cries-at-every-Hallmark-commercial wife took the biggest blow of all. We've gone through the same stages of grief—

denial, anger, depression, and begrudging acceptance—since that original day. Occasionally, we start all over again from the beginning when a new symptom appears or we hear of someone who is further along in the disease's progression.

That happened again recently when I met a few friends for lunch. One lady's husband had been suffering with Parkinson's for many years, and she gave us the latest update on his condition. She described how he had basically given up months before and succumbed to the depression he had been battling for years. He stopped doing any sort of exercise or physical therapy. He was now bedridden and unable to speak, and he rarely left his home. As a result, neither did she. Then she dropped the bombshell I don't think I'll ever be able to forget: "I just don't think he cared for or loved me enough to keep on trying. I guess I wasn't worth the effort."

I had no idea what to say. I think I muttered something about how that could not possibly be true, and it was probably just the depression talking. But I walked away from that conversation with a determination in my heart. I would do everything I possibly could to make sure such a thought never crossed Cheryl's mind. I want to make sure she knows that she is the main reason I want to not only survive but thrive. For her and our three daughters. And for the cutest grandson you've ever laid eyes on. I'm not just saying that, either. Complete strangers have confirmed it: Elisha's way cuter than your average grandson.

Here's what I want the world to know. While I still may feel guilty about being a burden, I'm so thankful that Cheryl is the one who God gave me to share my life with. I like to believe he led her to me, and I'm sure glad she was listening. May her hearing never fail! I know she will be there for me come hell or high water, no matter what may lie ahead for us. We've been through tough times together before, and, given the fact that we're rapidly approaching our thirtieth wedding anniversary, we do have a little bit of life experience already under our belt. Cheryl says they've been fifteen of the happiest years of her life. I'll let you do the math.

By now, you've probably noticed that we use a lot of humor in our relationship. It's one of our ways of handling whatever life may bring. But lest you think that all she ever does is offer snide remarks with perfect comedic timing, let me set the record straight: She is my "good thing." (See Proverbs 18:22.)

Cheryl is a beautiful woman, inside and out—the former being far more important, of course, but I can't really say I've minded the latter all these years. Her eyes will stop you in your tracks, and then melt your heart if you stand too close. I should know. I've been under their spell many times. She is intelligent and witty, and her laugh is absolutely contagious. She cries at the drop of a hat, and I mean any hat. She is the extrovert to my introvert. She is the fun factor to my moodiness. She is the quick-forgiver to my grudge-holding. She is the face I love to come home to, even without make-up, although I've never been able to convince her of that. I can only very rarely beat her at Five Crowns or Words With Friends, and I love that about her.

There are some things she cannot do well. She can't cook. She can't sing. She can't go for long periods of time without naps. She can't speak in public, or at least she doesn't like to. She can't lie very well, either—too many tell-tale signs. But once she's your friend, she's your friend for life. And there's not anything I would change about her. Well, except for her incessant watching of unsolved murder mysteries. I have to admit, that one does make me nervous at times, especially when she's taking notes. I'm sure that's not significant in any way. I just chalk it up to her wanting to be a lifelong learner. Right, Hon?

~

So, let me dedicate the next few pages to the love of my life. If this gets too mushy for anyone, please feel free to skip this part. That'd be totally understandable. But the truth is that those of us with Parkinson's owe a great debt to our care partners. And as I gaze ahead into the unknown, there are some hopes and promises that I want to share with mine. This is my Parkinson's Partner Pledge, if you will, that I intend to honor for as long as I have the mental and/or physical capacity to do so. Here's what I pledge:

1. I plan to prove to you every day that I believe you *are* worth it. How? I will never stop trying, never stop fighting, and never stop using all my strength and willpower to beat this thing. I don't want there to ever be even the smallest doubt in your heart and mind of how much you mean to me.

2. I plan to tell you and show you in as many ways as possible how much I love you. I am determined to keep on whispering those words in your ear every morning, dancing with you in the kitchen every afternoon, and holding your hand in bed every night. In other words: same old, same old for us.

3. I plan to always say thank you for the things you do for me and never take you for granted. I hope I'm getting both of those things right even now in our relationship, but I feel it's even more imperative for me to do so going forward. May you see in my eyes and hear in my voice that I am truly grateful.

4. I plan to do my best to be sensitive to and aware of your needs, wants, and dreams. I don't ever want this whole thing to become just about me. How boring would that be? Your needs are just as important as mine, and I hope to never let that truth get lost in the shuffle for either one of us. Pun intended.

5. I plan to never lose my sense of humor, and I don't want you to ever lose yours. We've used that effective "medicine" throughout all these years of marriage, parenting, and just doing life together. Whatever comes next, may we both keep on laughing, especially at ourselves.

6. I plan to guard against overburdening you with my needs to the point that you feel stressed out or burnt out. If this should ever become 24/7, we're going to make a way for you to escape when you need to—to spend time with family or friends, enjoy some quiet moments alone, or maybe just take a nap. I know how you feel about naps.

7. I hope to continue to be able to serve you in big ways and small ways. We both know that "acts of service" has always been my love language. If I'm fearful of losing any ability in the future, it's that one. I may have to get more creative in the days ahead, but I will find a way, I promise.

8. I hope to forgive quickly and keep short accounts in all my relationships, but especially with you. You're actually the one who has taught me that over the years—to come out of my man cave sooner rather than later and to let go of my grudges for the sake of my own heart. May the sun never go down while we are still angry. Or while I am, right?

9. I hope to face this whole journey without any unnecessary anxiety or fear in our hearts. Worry will never add a single hour to our lives. Or as you like to say, "Sufficient unto the day is the evil, thereof." May we learn to take everything that comes our way one day at a time.

10. Lastly, I hope never to cause you to lose faith or doubt God for anything that has happened or will happen to me. You know how I feel about all this: God can heal me, and he still may, but even if he does not, I trust him to give me the grace I need to make it through. I'm praying he gives you that same grace.

There are probably other things I should pledge, I know, but I think ten is a good number with which to start. After all, God had his top ten in the Old Testament, right? But a funny thing happened on the way to the New Testament. Jesus was once asked which commandment was the greatest, and he responded that there were basically two that summed up all the rest: Love God with all your heart, soul, mind, and strength; and love your neighbor as yourself—which brings us right back to where we started ... Galatians 5: "Serve one another humbly in love. For the entire law is fulfilled in keeping this one command: 'Love your neighbor as yourself.'" To all who love someone with Parkinson's and for those of us with Parkinson's who love them in return, let those words be the motto and mantra of our lives.

HABITUDES

Do you not know that in a race all the runners run, but only one gets the prize? Run in such a way as to get the prize. Everyone who competes in the games goes into strict training. They do it to get a crown that will not last, but we do it to get a crown that will last forever. Therefore I do not run like someone running aimlessly; I do not fight like a boxer beating the air. No, I strike a blow to my body and make it my slave so that ... I myself will not be disqualified for the prize.
—1 Corinthians 9:24-27

You know that I'm a teacher, but I'm in the classroom much less now that I'm also an assistant principal. I do miss the daily interaction with the students. They still come by often to see me, mind you, but nowadays it's not always for positive reasons. For several years prior, though, my main assignment was teaching the four high school Bible classes. No, it's not a public school. How did you know?

I've also taught a leadership class for upperclassmen for the last two years, which I have thoroughly enjoyed. The main feature of the course was to take the students to interview leaders in our own community, from the mayor of the city to the pastor of a nearby megachurch, from a local judge to the recently announced teacher of the year, from the

CEO of one of the two healthcare systems in town to the chairperson of our area's United Way. There's nothing like letting proven leaders talk to our students about real world leadership. I loved that they were able to go beyond just a written curriculum.

However, we did talk theory as well during the weeks that we did not take one of our field trips. I tried using different resources for the lecture and discussion portion of the course, but I didn't hit pay dirt until I found a series of books on leadership created by Tim Elmore of Growing Leaders, based out of Norcross, Georgia. The series is called *Habitudes®: Images that Form Leadership Habits and Attitudes.* What I thought was so innovative about the series is that it was primarily image driven; that is, each leadership principle was tied to a full-color photograph that helped engrave the idea in the hearts and minds of the students. (Visit GrowingLeaders.com for more information.) It was a fantastic way to teach on leadership.

I also just like the word *habitudes*, that perfect blend between the two ideas of habits and attitudes that were essential to my leadership class but perhaps even more so to my struggle with Parkinson's. My doctor spelled it out from the beginning: I had a chronic disease that for some people was debilitating, but for many people it was merely a nuisance, annoying at worst. If I'm lucky enough to be in the latter category, much would depend on me, he had explained. I would need to think in the right ways and do the right things, and then make those thoughts and practices part of my daily routine. My habits would help create the proper attitudes within me, and then those very attitudes would help inspire the appropriate habits. And so a virtuous cycle would begin and continue to positively reinforce itself, ideally leading to a completely new way of living. Diagnoses change the way people live all the time. My diagnosis would do the same for me.

~

In 1 Corinthians 9, the Apostle Paul alludes to the Isthmian Games of Corinth that took place every other year as the backdrop of an important point he was trying to communicate. The Isthmian Games were almost as popular as the ones held in Olympia every four years, but we know now which of the two ancient Greek cities had the better ad agency. Sportscasters all over the world are probably very happy today that the Isthmic Games didn't win out, unless they enjoy speaking with a lisp.

For the sake of his Corinthian readers, however, I'm sure that Paul didn't even mention that *other* competition when he described the preparation and performance of the athletes who participated in the games: "Do you not know that in a race all the runners run, but only one gets the prize? Run in such a way as to get the prize. Everyone who competes in the games goes into strict training. They do it to get a crown that will not last, but we do it to get a crown that will last forever" (1 Corinthians 9:24-25). That last line tells us that Paul is ultimately talking about a spiritual truth: Just as the great athletes disciplined themselves in order to win the prize—which was in those days a woven wreath made out of either dried celery, pine needles or olive branches—so the followers of Christ would need to discipline themselves in order to finish well and gain a crown of a little more enduring substance and significance.

He concludes the passage by picturing himself as one of the competitors in the games: "Therefore I do not run like someone running aimlessly; I do not fight like a boxer beating the air. No, I strike a blow to my body and make it my slave so that … I myself will not be disqualified for the prize" (1 Corinthians 9:26-27). Essentially, Paul says, whatever it takes to win the prize, that's what I will do. I will discipline both my body and my mind to make sure that happens. Body and mind. Habits and attitudes. Habitudes.

~

If you're looking for a peer-reviewed and medically sound list of action steps that a person with Parkinson's might follow that have been clinically proven to stave off or deter the progress of the disease, then this chapter is not for you. Instead, I would like to share what I have been doing personally for the health of both my body and mind. There are no magic formulas here. Each of us must discover what works for our version of Parkinson's and what distinguishes a good day from a bad day. I'm going to talk about six habitudes that I have made part of my daily regimen. And should I leave out any one of them on a given day, I have found that I will suffer the consequences: increased visibility of the motor symptoms and an acute awareness of the non-motor symptoms, including depression and irritability.

My wife, Cheryl, always sees the difference immediately and will invariably ask, "Did you take your pills?" To which I will respond either kindly or not so kindly, depending on whether or not I took my pills. Or put into practice these habitudes.

~

I think the biggest change for me has been my diet, mainly because the other five habitudes were things I was already doing in my life but now they had just become even more important for me. My nutritional intake, however, needed some adjustment, and it was my diagnosis that helped me to finally see the truth. The actual wake-up call came when I visited my primary care doctor for an annual physical, and he noticed that my weight had ballooned. I told him I had noticed that as well and that it was all due to the Parkinson's. I walk slower now, I patiently explained to him, so I get less exercise within the same period of time.

He looked at me for half a second before responding: "Parkinson's has nothing to do with it. McDonald's maybe, but not Parkinson's." Did I tell you that he's not as compassionate and jovial as my neurologist? He continued: "You'll never get the weight down just by exercising. Walk three miles, and you'll barely take off a granola bar. What you need to do is reduce your calorie intake, pure and simple." He suggested that I start keeping a food diary, which I did ... and then burned it. The truth of those pages shall never again be seen by human eyes, but it did begin the process of helping me to think correctly in this one area of my life.

When I later told a friend of mine about how rude the doctor had been, he suggested that I get over it and check out an online food diary that he had discovered, and, thus, my new nutritional life began. (See myfitnesspal.com for more information.) Incredibly, I immediately dropped twenty pounds, and that was simply because I had become more aware of what I was consuming. I started the plan primarily for the weight loss benefit, and it has certainly helped me achieve that, but the by-product has been that I am much more conscious of which foods are healthy for me and which foods are not. I can still overindulge at times, but I have found that having to write it all down helps to curb my cravings. I may even still swing through McDonald's every now and again, but now I know what to order off the menu that will not blow my calorie count for the whole day. In addition, the plan also asks me to record the number of glasses of water I drink every day, something else I had been negligent about. That's not true, anymore.

The fantastic thing about all this is that eating healthier has caused me to feel healthier which translates into more energy, less fatigue, better self-esteem, and even the occasional wolf whistle from my wife, all of which lead me to continue the new dietary habits. It's that virtuous cycle I described earlier, with the encouraging feedback loop built in, especially the whistle.

~

Exercise is the second habitude, which I'm sure you

probably could have guessed. Eating right and staying active are the key to so many health problems, both in their prevention and treatment. Diet and exercise obviously help with issues like obesity, diabetes, and coronary heart disease, but numerous studies also suggest that they can dramatically improve the quality of life of those with everything from cancer to dementia and, yes, even Parkinson's. My neurologist told me early on that exercise would not increase the amount of dopamine in my brain, nor would it regrow the brain cells that had already degenerated, but it would potentially help decrease significantly the frequency and intensity of my visible symptoms. Exercise is to the Parkinson's brain, he said, what motor oil is to the engine of a car. It lubricates and helps all the working parts function together more smoothly, without locking up. I'd settle for that.

I already had a regular routine of exercising every day. I've always been too cheap to pay for a gym membership but I did have a dog that needed to be walked every morning, so usually before sunrise the two of us would walk a block and then jog a block for a total of three miles or forty-five minutes, whichever came first. Then the symptoms began, and we got the shocking news of the diagnosis. Somewhere during that time, I confess that I went through a period of depression that all but wiped out that daily routine.

But once the meds began to help stabilize the symptoms, I realized that walking first thing in the morning helped produce a fluidity of motion that carried over into rest of the day. It was like spraying WD-40 on a rusty hinge: The more you spray, the more freedom of movement you're able to see. Skipping a morning or two of walking had the opposite effect, and the difference was dramatic. So, I have made it my practice to walk at least thirty minutes every morning, longer if there's time. At work, I take the stairs and not the elevator, and I leave my office frequently to talk with my colleagues rather than email them or use the two-way radio. I believe that every step helps.

Sometimes, I do push-ups, lift hand weights and

occasionally work through the exercises my physical therapist taught me as part of my BIG™ training—a variety of multidirectional movements that are specifically designed to increase the ease and range of movement in my torso and limbs. I call them the *ta-da* exercises because they tend to include exaggerated motions in which I appear to be taking a bow, or I'm stretching my hands and fingers as far as they will go toward the ceiling and then the floor, or I'm extending first one arm and then the other out in front of me as if I am presenting the next act. It's hard for me not to say, "*Ta-da!*" after each rep.

I believe the secret to exercise is finding an activity that results in a measurable difference in your day and yet is not so unappealing that you avoid it for whatever excuse you can dream up. It must be something that you will enjoy enough to continue doing and that your doctor would approve of you doing. The latest crazes in my part of the country are gentle yoga, tai chi, and dance classes. I haven't tried those, yet, but I'm willing. Bring on the WD-40!

~

The next habitude may seem to contradict the previous one, but it's just as important. It's sleep or rest. This is my wife's favorite habitude. By her own description, she is neither a morning person nor a night owl, and she has the amazing ability to take a lengthy nap on a weekend afternoon and still go to bed early that evening. I like to tease that her best hours of the day are between ten and two. She tells me I'm just jealous—which may be partially true—and quotes Psalm 127:2 to me: "He grants sleep to those he loves."

Over the last two years, my sleep quotient has made a huge difference in my Parkinson's day. If I don't get enough rest, the fatigue factor creates the opposite of the virtuous cycle in me, the more infamous vicious cycle. I wake up shuffling heavily, my meds don't seem to kick in as quickly or as efficiently as usual, I skip my morning walk because I simply don't feel like it, and the rest of the day is, in a word, sluggish. That kind of snowball effect may be true of all human beings after too little sleep, but I think it's amplified in people with Parkinson's. Our bodies and brains just need more time to be refreshed. And sadly, there are all kinds of sleep disorders that are associated with Parkinson's, everything from insomnia to restless leg syndrome to central sleep apnea, which occurs when the brain fails to send the right signals to the muscles that control a person's breathing. Sound familiar? Coincidentally, I was diagnosed with sleep apnea several years before the Parkinson's diagnosis. My neurologist said it was probably an early sign of what was coming.

Now, I'm almost fanatical about getting enough hours of rest so that I don't start the day already behind. I used to get by on four or five hours of sleep, but those days are gone forever. Now, I shoot for at least seven or eight every night, except for those rare occasions when I find myself in unusual circumstances like, for instance, writing a book. Who knew writers sometimes get up in the middle of the night feeling inspired to type out another thousand words or so? But don't worry, I'm in good hands. I now have a sleep therapist who is quite the trained professional. In fact, I'm married to her.

~

So, we should eat right, exercise, and get plenty of rest. Almost any doctor in the world would have suggested those three things, no matter what the disease or medical condition. The next three habitudes, however, are less prescribed officially, but I'm quite sure that they are just as important. At least, they have been for me. They're activities and mindsets that I was already practicing before my D-Day. I just happen to feel even more strongly about them now.

The first of the final three is reading. I'm a voracious reader. I'm convinced that one of the ways I'm keeping my mind sharp, focused, and off the negativity of my circumstances is by continuing to explore the magnificent world of words and all the beauty, truth, and imagination they invoke. And when I say read, I mean every day and every opportunity you get. I mean turning off the televisions and computer monitors and getting lost in the pages of a moving story, a momentous time in history, or a theological treatise on a neurodegenerative disease. I may have lost you on that last one, but my point is that you're always starting, in the middle of, or finishing up the latest book, and the next one is on the coffee table waiting its turn.

I grew up in a family of readers, so I'm biased. I realize that. But this habitude really kicked in about sixteen years ago when an esteemed colleague of mine challenged me to start a book log of my reading journey as a way of developing myself personally and professionally. "Leaders are readers," he said, "and they never stop learning." So, that year I read twelve and felt great about the new endeavor. "You should double that," he remarked when I gave him the count, and so I did, plus twenty-eight more. *That should quiet him*, I thought. But instead, he smiled and commented, "Now you can never go back." And it was true. It has become such an ingrained habit that I've hit fifty-two almost every year since. I have not regretted a single moment. I still prefer the print versions, but I like the electronic versions when I travel. And I do have my favorite authors, but I force myself to read not just the genres I enjoy but also many that stretch me intellectually, emotionally, and spiritually, as well. My lists include everything from best-selling novels and self-help books to biographies and the sometimes-thick texts required for my unending graduate classes. The last couple of years have included multiple titles that have something to do with Parkinson's disease.

I read once that doing mind puzzles such as the crossword and Sudoku every day helped to deter, or at least decrease, the chances of dementia. I think I remember seeing later that this idea was debunked. I'm not sure which is true, but I do know this: Reading and educating your mind

definitely does not prevent Parkinson's. If that were true,
you'd think that I would have a clean bill of health. It has
been an effective coping mechanism for me, however, and
therapeutic to my mind and my heart. There's even a fancy
word for all this, *bibliotherapy*. You should read more about it.

~

   The next habitude that is a big part of my life is
volunteering. Specifically, I'm talking about when we serve,
assist, or in some way help those who are less fortunate than
we are. If you will remember, we've said that the Parkinson's
brain tends toward smallness—small steps, small motions,
etc. I would say that our brains also tend toward inwardness.
Physically, I've seen it in a symptom called *dystonia*, which is
when the fingers and toes and sometimes even the feet
themselves curl inward, almost like a claw. One of my
constant exercises is to just stretch my fingers and toes as far
outward as I can to combat that tendency. I can sense that
same inclination at times mentally, as well, on those days
when it seems like it would be so much easier just to stay
home and isolate myself from all human contact rather than
fight through the awkwardness of my symptoms yet another
day. But just as I stretch out my fingers, I also stretch out my
soul, if you will.
   I intentionally look for ways to get out and serve others
so that I'm not just focusing on me and my problems. That's
why I volunteered to help with our local Parkinson
Association of the Carolinas the very next day after meeting
the executive director. My thinking? I'm new to Parkinson's,
and the disease is only in the early stages for me. There are so
many people farther along than I am that I could potentially
help and serve. My Parkinson's buddy, Vince, and I are
making plans now to help restart a support group in our area.
We are deliberately moving outward, not inward.
   For the last ten years or so, I have also volunteered at a
breakfast for the homeless, served every Sunday morning in

downtown Charlotte. The guys who started this ministry have not missed a Sunday in more than fifteen years. We set up tables and chairs outside every week and start dishing out the hot eggs, grits, and sausage at six-thirty sharp. We typically serve between one hundred and two hundred men and women who either live on the streets or in the nearby shelters.

When I first started helping, the workers were few, and I was behind the tables most weeks spooning out the eggs or grits, or filling up cups with juice, milk, or coffee. The ministry has gained a little more popularity in recent years, however, and now we have plenty of helpers. So, I moved out from behind the tables, and I stand each week at the beginning of the line, where I can warmly greet each person with a handshake or a pat on the back and simply say, "Welcome. Enjoy the breakfast!" I'm convinced that for some of them, it might be one of the few positive words or physical touches they receive all week.

Some of the men and women have been coming to the breakfast so often that we know one another by name. Occasionally, I have been downtown during the week on a field trip and one of my homeless acquaintances will come over to hug me and greet me by name. My students, after they get over the shock, think that's about the coolest thing in the world. It gives me street cred, I think they call it. The thing that I think is so cool is that none of those men and women from the breakfast know that I have Parkinson's. I'm just the nice guy who smiles at them as they arrive and ushers them into our makeshift restaurant on the street. Sunday mornings are not about me, it's about them, and that's the way it should be. But whether they realize it or not, they're helping me, as well—to think outwardly, not inwardly. I plan to keep moving in that direction.

~

The final habitude that keeps me focused on the right

things is to make sure that I love those around me completely and fully. There's something about learning that you have an incurable disease that makes you rethink your priorities. Now, don't get me wrong. I'm taking my doctor's word that many people with Parkinson's live long and productive lives. They just have to deal with those annoying little symptoms that seem to tag along. So, for the sake of my three daughters who will almost certainly read these words, I don't think I'm dying or anything. Don't get all weepy. (Your mom will do that for all of us.) But there is a song Tim McGraw made famous a few years ago that often goes through my mind.

The title was "Live Like You Were Dying"—written by Tim Nichols and Craig Wiseman—and the words are of a man who finds out that he has come to the end of his life and he's asked what he did when he heard the news. And, evidently, he begins singing at the top of his lungs about skydiving, mountain climbing, and bull riding; none of which, I can assure you, would come to my mind if I received the same verdict. Nothing personal, Fu Man Chu. But there is one line from the chorus I can never get out of my head. If you're a country music fan, you probably know which one it is. The dying man speaks to my soul when he says: "And I loved deeper, and I spoke sweeter, and I gave forgiveness I'd been denying." That's exactly what I mean when I talk about the habitude of loving. Life is too fleeting and fragile to waste a single moment. I said it from the very beginning. When you realize every day is a gift, you tend to focus on the things that really matter. You tend to focus on the *people* who really matter. You use every second you've been given wisely, ideally with everyone you meet, but especially with your family and friends. You learn to give love and receive it in return.

One of the ways my family and I have tried to do that is by discovering one another's love language. If that sounds totally unfamiliar to you, the concept is based on a book by Gary Chapman entitled *The Five Love Languages*, and his essential premise is that we all have a particular means through which we express our love to others and by which we prefer that others express their love to us. Briefly, the five "languages" are words of affirmation, quality time, receiving gifts, acts of service, and physical touch. (Check out his website at 5lovelanguages.com for more information.)

I know, for instance, that I show love through acts of service, a fact to which all my girls can attest. But I feel loved through words of affirmation—verbal encouragement and compliments. That sounds so shallow as I type out those words, but Cheryl says I'm not at all shallow, but rather a very witty, intelligent, and charming middle-aged man. She has such a way with words.

All five ways are legitimate means to express your feelings for someone else, but knowing which language speaks to that person the most effectively is an enhancement to any relationship. When I do premarital counseling for young couples, I always recommend that they become linguistic experts before the end of their sessions with me. The ones that follow my advice have a definite advantage going forward. They can love deeper and speak sweeter from the very start.

This habitude of loving, in short, means I make sure that those whom I love know it and there's no shadow of a doubt in their minds about where they stand with me. It means that I live each day with little or no regrets in my relationships, as much as that is humanly possible, listening more than I talk, and thinking before I speak. So many interpersonal problems could be solved by those two simple actions alone. To love means that I don't get angry or take offense easily and that I'm quick to forgive, not allowing even the hint of bitterness to fester and poison my heart. To love means that I look for and believe in the best in others and that I maintain a somewhat selective memory, editing out the parts that are not worth retaining and recording forever the parts that I definitely want to be included on the highlight reel. This is the habitude more than any of the others that I want to get right.

~

Am I really saying that reading books, volunteering to serve the less fortunate, and loving those around us will diminish the effects of Parkinson's on our lives? Well, yes, but only because those kinds of activities are all part of living well in general and help make us the right sort of people. And if we can say those things are true of our lives, then we are living well with Parkinson's, too. It hasn't beaten us. In fact, it may actually be the reason that we try even harder to get life right.

In the 1 Corinthians passage we looked at earlier, Paul admonishes us to run in such a way as to get the prize. Go into strict training, he says, and discipline yourselves in order that you will not be disqualified. The prize he was referring to was a crown in heaven, given by none other than God himself to those who finish well. Looking at the end of his life, to the last words he ever penned, this is what Paul was able to say to his young protégé, Timothy: "The time for my departure is near. I have fought the good fight, I have finished the race, I have kept the faith. Now there is in store for me the crown of righteousness, which the Lord, the righteous Judge, will award to me on that day—and not only to me, but also to all who have longed for his appearing" (2 Timothy 4:6-8). He got the prize.

The habitudes that I've mentioned in this chapter are my own disciplines that help me finish well this race of life I'm running, regardless of the Parkinson's. My challenge to you is to do the same. You may even come up with your own set of habitudes that mold you into the person that you want to become. I believe that's worth doing, whether you have Parkinson's or not.

HEART

Above all else, guard your heart, for everything you do flows from it.
—Proverbs 4:23

I've admired Michael J. Fox for many years, both as an award-winning actor and more recently as a spokesperson, if not *the* spokesperson, for the disease we share. At the time of this writing, Michael was diagnosed some twenty-two years ago. I barely made it under the wire at the age of forty-nine when it comes to the diagnosis of young onset Parkinson's. Michael deserves his title—he was only twenty-nine years old when he first got the news and made national headlines. Yet, he has done so much for the cause of Parkinson's since that day. He has been very busy. His foundation, cleverly titled The Michael J. Fox Foundation, has raised over $350 million to help with the treatment of the disease, as well as the research to find a cure. I have to admit: I'm rooting for him with all my heart.

Cheryl and I recently saw Michael on the David Letterman Show. It was disheartening to watch him struggle with *dyskinesia* as he sat in the chair next to David's desk. These jerky, repetitive movements are a side effect of the medications many of us take for Parkinson's—*not* of the disease itself. I looked over and watched Cheryl weep silently. I reminded her that this was not necessarily my future, that every journey was unique.

To which she responded, "I'm not crying." She's such a terrible liar.

But there was one thing about the interview that I found absolutely amazing. I'm not sure where Michael J. Fox might see himself in religious or spiritual terms, but his response to one of David Letterman's questions sounded downright biblical and resonated with so much of what I've been saying throughout these pages. I'm not sure if it was scripted, as so many of those late night talks are, but Letterman seemed to start one question and then abruptly asked Michael off the cuff: "Do you ever sometimes think that this is the way life works, that had you not been diagnosed that Parkinson's would not be this much farther along in raising money for research and treatment?"

To which Michael gave this remarkable reply: "I don't think about that too much. I look at this as a real opportunity and a privilege. And really I'm happy I was put in this, I mean, I truly am happy that I was put in this situation because I have so many opportunities and resources to push research along. It's just one of those things. It's like I always say. It's been a gift that keeps on taking ... but it's been a gift."

I recorded the interview and replayed it several times to make sure I was hearing his words correctly, mainly because I was floored at the kind of language he used. With genuine humility, he deflected the question about the money he had raised and instead talked about how he viewed his Parkinson's as an opportunity, a privilege, and a gift. It sounded like something a pastor might say, and I know fairly well what that sounds like. Cheryl, who was still not crying, agreed with me. It felt like Michael was speaking from the heart at that moment and, if so, it was an enlightening glimpse into his soul.

The whole evening got me reflecting on what I would say if I spoke from my heart. I think I would probably say some of the same things he said, at least publicly. But the question that wouldn't go away, even after we turned off the television and headed for bed, was: Is that what I truly believe deep down in my heart? When it's just me and God, and no one else can hear, what would my soul say?

~

Solomon was the wisest man who ever lived, at least according to the Bible. If you don't know his story, he was the son of King David, the giant-killer, and Bathsheba, whose name is certainly appropriate when you read about how she and the king actually met. That's a tale for another time and place. But however scandalous the union between his mom and dad had been, Solomon was chosen to succeed his father as the king of Israel.

As he was about to begin his reign, God appeared to him in a dream and said, "Ask for whatever you want me to give you" (1 Kings 3:5). It's not really the best offer to make to a young man about to become the richest, most powerful man in the known world. But Solomon showed restraint and humbly asked for a discerning heart and the ability to distinguish between right and wrong so that he would be a good king who governed his people well.

And 1 Kings 3:10-13 reports that God was pleased with this request and responds, "OK, I'll give you what you asked for—a wise and discerning heart. Moreover [which is a word that only sounds correct if God is saying it], I will give you what you have not asked for—wealth and honor and a long life." The whole scenario seems to point to the fact that Solomon had a little bit of wisdom coming in to his position, even before he made his noble request of God.

His first real test comes when two prostitutes appear before him with an infant, both claiming to be the baby's mother. After listening to their stories, he calls for a sword and orders that the child be cut in two so that half could be given to one mother and half to the other. On the surface, it doesn't exactly sound like the wisdom has kicked in, yet. But then one mom steps forward and asks that the baby not be killed but instead be given to the other woman, and Solomon immediately knows that she is the real mother.

When the kingdom hears about the verdict, the Bible says that everyone was in awe of the king's wisdom, except perhaps for the baby, who, upon hearing the tale later in life, probably thought that there might have been a better way to get to the truth. But the news of Solomon's wisdom quickly spread far and wide, and people from all over the world came just to hear him talk. And it was this same Solomon the Wise who wrote the words that begin this chapter: "Above all else, guard your heart for everything you do flows from it." Wise words, indeed.

I do feel, however, that I should mention one caveat regarding Solomon's wisdom. The Bible also says that he had seven hundred wives and three hundred concubines *and* that he published a famous love poem to just *one* of them. I'm thinking they probably didn't call him Solomon the Wise back at the castle for a while. In fact, there are some indications that he might have had to sleep on the roof for a few days. (See Proverbs 21:9 and 25:24.) My point is that he evidently had some blind spots when it came to wise ways.

But Solomon did get it right, I believe, with these words that we're focusing on, because Jesus said something very similar in the New Testament that corroborates them. In Luke 6, Jesus is teaching his disciples a truth about the heart. He says: "No good tree bears bad fruit, nor does a bad tree bear good fruit. Each tree is recognized by its own fruit. People do not pick figs from thornbushes, or grapes from briers. A good man brings good things out of the good stored up in his heart, and an evil man brings evil things out of the evil stored up in his heart. For the mouth speaks what the heart is full of" (Luke 6:43-45). Wow, I don't know how many times I've thought that last line.

But let me emphasize that both Solomon and Jesus say that our heart is the wellspring out of which the rest of our life flows. We're not talking about the organ that pumps the blood through the circulatory system, but instead that part of us that is the center, or the innermost core, of our being.

And Jesus made it very clear: A good heart produces good things. A bad heart, not so much. What's the key? What makes the difference? You have to protect the originating spring from which the whole river emanates. Merely cleaning up downstream won't do you much good in the long run if the spring itself is contaminated. You have to guard the source, Solomon said. You have to guard the heart.

~

One of the first things my neurologist warned me to watch for was depression. In fact, either he or a member of his staff asks me about it at some point during almost every visit. I think at first they were just checking on how I was handling the news of the diagnosis. With time, the questions had more to do with my reaction to the medications I was taking. In fact, every time we adjusted the dosages, they could be counted on like clockwork to check up on me, either by calling me or asking me to call them.

I remember once, after we had increased the prescribed amount for one of my meds, the head nurse for my neurologist called a few days later to check on whether I had had any side effects since the change. She inquired specifically about depression, hallucinations, and any suicidal thoughts. I told her I was doing OK on all fronts. Then, just as we were about to end the call, she suddenly thought of one more thing: "Oh, and sometimes this medicine can produce compulsive behaviors. Have you had any of those?"

"Like what?" I asked.

"Like a sudden urge to go shopping or start gambling, things like that," she replied.

I deadpanned: "I wish you had called a little sooner. I

lost our house last night in a poker game. We had to move in with my in-laws."

She half-scolded, "I should have known not to worry about you," and hung up the phone, laughing.

But I'm glad she does worry. Depression, and other non-motor symptoms and side effects associated with Parkinson's and its various forms of treatment, can be serious business. It is estimated that that at least half of all Parkinson's patients suffer from clinical depression, which means that it's severe enough that they need to be treated. For the right treatment to take place, though, the medical caregivers have to be made aware of the problem. It's almost impossible to spot things like depression, apathy, or anxiety during an occasional doctor visit. The patients themselves, or the people who know them best, need to report what they are feeling or seeing.

I believe a big part of guarding your heart is to be self-aware enough to notice your own emotions, reactions, and feelings, and when you see a downturn, be courageous enough to ask for help. You may require additional medication; or it might be necessary to visit a certified counselor, psychiatrist, or psychologist. Sometimes, you can turn the corner with the help of a Parkinson's support group or by talking with your pastor or spiritual advisor. The main thing is to know you need help and then ask for it.

I saw a billboard a few months ago that simply said, "This year, thousands of men will die from stubbornness." My wife, sensing that I was about to say something in defense of men everywhere, reached over, patted my leg, and said, "Prove it wrong." I hate it when she wins the argument before I even say the first word.

~

We have to recognize that sometimes our heart issues—depression, anxiety, and the like—are actually medical conditions that need to be treated. However, if that diagnosis is ruled out, we also need to consider the possibility that often the optimism or pessimism we feel is a decision that we willfully make in our own hearts. To say it another way, we choose whether we're going to see the glass half empty or half full, whether we're going to give up or keep fighting, and whether we're going to focus on the negative or be able to see the positive in the midst of it all.

Back when Ronald Reagan was president, he was known for his humor and wit, often disarming his opponents with a well-timed punch line. He reportedly had a favorite joke, though, that he shared whenever he got the opportunity. It went something like this: The parents of a little boy thought their son was a little too optimistic, so they took him to see a psychiatrist. Trying to bring him down a notch or two, the psychiatrist took him into a room piled high with horse manure. Yet, instead of displaying disgust, the little boy climbed to the top of the pile and began digging excitedly. The psychiatrist was flabbergasted.

"What in the world are you doing?" he yelled above the boy's enthusiastic screams. "Why are you digging?"

The boy looked down beaming and said, "Because with all this manure, there must be a pony in here somewhere."

Now that's being optimistic, wouldn't you agree? And I know it's just a joke, but doesn't it seem a tad bit foolish as well?

I want to be clear that what I'm advocating here is not some Pollyanna approach to life that is blindly hopeful and always obnoxiously cheerful. Those kinds of people are just as exasperating to me as they are to everyone else on the planet, especially when they happen to be morning people, as well. Solomon the Wise agreed. Here's what he wrote in Proverbs 27:14, another verse that I bet you didn't know was in the Bible: "If anyone loudly blesses their neighbor early in the morning, it will be taken as a curse." It would appear that even God dislikes morning people.

No, what I'm suggesting is that, while we must never refuse to see the reality of our circumstances, we shouldn't allow ourselves to get mired down in the negative. Yes, we need to acknowledge our difficulties and concede that we have limitations that we didn't have before. But then we optimistically move forward anyway, which is the only direction we can go. We either stagnate or we move ahead. The only thing we can't do is go back.

So, the question becomes: Will we take the next step with hope or with despair? It can often be a matter of the heart, for it's in our hearts that we decide if we're going to stop trying or keep fighting. It's in our hearts that we choose to emphasize what we can't do or focus instead on the things we can still do, and then go and do them. The decisions we make deep down in our innermost being flow out and become the words and actions of our lives.

~

I remember the first time I experienced the symptom called *dystonia* in my feet. I was on my morning walk and quite a distance from our townhouse. Without warning, my toes started curling inward, and in time my whole right foot did the same. My foot wouldn't uncurl, and I was literally standing on the side of my foot and in a good bit of pain. I hobbled home and left a voice message for my neurologist reporting what happened. Later, he called and confirmed that I was dealing with yet another not-so-rare symptom of Parkinson's. I was devastated. I love my morning walks. They set the tone for the rest of my day. This was going to seriously cramp my style.

I had a couple of good days in a row with no symptoms, but then about a week later, it happened again. I was at least a half-mile from home. I almost called Cheryl to come get me but instead decided that I was not going to allow this new development to take away my primary means of exercise. I started experimenting with ways to correct my gait. I first considered tying a belt or rope to my foot and lifting it by hand for each step. For those who do not have Parkinson's, I know that sounds ridiculous, but that's the nature of the disease. A person has to sometimes make the body do what the brain usually handles. The nearest belt or rope was at the house, however, so that wasn't going to work.

Then I looked down at the curb and had an ingenious idea. I started walking again, gingerly, except this time I let my left foot land in the road—which only worked because I live in a quiet suburban community with very little traffic—and I let my right foot come down on the curb itself. With each step, I caught the top of the curb with my toes and the curvature of the concrete forced the rest of my foot to extend and unfold. Now, mind you, I did look silly walking down the road, stepping up and down, up and down, as if one leg were shorter than the other. But I was walking at five-thirty in the morning, so who was going to notice? The important thing is that it worked. Later, my doctor would adjust my meds and the frequency of that particular symptom decreased, although it has not completely gone away.

But what I took away from the incident was that I could do one of two things when I faced an obstacle related to my Parkinson's. First, I could wallow in my own self-pity and write off some of my favorite activities in the process—much too easily, in my opinion. Or I could look beyond the difficulties and search instead for ways to beat the problems. The obstacle would still be there, but my reaction to it would make all the difference. I would look for a pony in there somewhere.

I can say that my symptoms have affected many different areas of my life: walking, sleeping, sitting, typing, reading, remembering, shaving, showering, even talking. Cheryl often feels the need to finish my sentences. Of course, she's always done that, so it's a little hard to measure. The bottom line is, I've had to make this decision to push ahead quite a few times at this point. And as much as it depends on me, I'm going to continue to opt for optimism.

~

History tells us that Martha Dandridge Custis Washington, the wife of George Washington, the first president of the United States, did not like the limelight that came with her husband's political position. She would have much more preferred to return to their home, Mount Vernon. But a new nation had been born and duty called. When her husband decided to answer that call, Martha was faced with her own decision: either give in to resentment and depression over being away from home or make a choice to be content with her present circumstances, no matter what they might be.

During her time as the first First Lady, she wrote these words to a friend: "I am still determined to be cheerful and happy, in whatever situation I may be; for I have also learned from experience that the greater part of our happiness or misery depends upon our dispositions, and not upon our circumstances."

"Our *dispositions*," she says. Often, when we use that term, we are referring to the way our minds are inclined to think about certain things. Some people believe that we are born with a particular disposition or temperament. I think that is partially true. But I also believe that we learn many of our behaviors and our reactions to whatever life throws at us, based on our personal walks through life. Nature *and* nurture make us who we are. When Martha writes, "I am determined to be cheerful and happy," it sounds like something that may not have felt natural for her in the circumstances she faced, but she was resolute in her decision. She would be cheerful and happy, no matter what.

The Apostle Paul uses almost the exact same wording in his letter to the Philippians. When the believers at Philippi sent him a missionary offering to further his church planting efforts, he sends them a thank you epistle. He expresses his gratitude, but then he talks about what he had *learned* to do when facing both good and bad circumstances:

I rejoiced greatly in the Lord that at last you renewed
your concern for me. Indeed, you were concerned, but
you had no opportunity to show it. I am not saying this
because I am in need, for I have learned to be content
whatever the circumstances. I know what it is to be in
need, and I know what it is to have plenty. I have learned
the secret of being content in any and every situation,
whether well fed or hungry, whether living in plenty or in
want. I can do all this through him who gives me
strength (Philippians 4:10-13).

In Christian circles, we so often use that last line out of
context, psyching ourselves up to climb a mountain, give a
speech, or get a job. I know God can help you with all those
things, but what Paul was specifically talking about here was
his ability to do what he had just described—to live through
feast or famine, stuffed belly or starving, good or bad. Those
were the "all things" he could do through Christ who gave
him strength. And the reason God had to give him strength
was because what he was proposing did not come naturally to
him, or to any of us, for that matter. It was something that he
had to learn to do—that was his part in the equation—but it
was also something that he needed help to accomplish—that
was God's part.

I can't move on without diving into the context of these
verses a little more. As I said earlier in this book, if you're not
from a religious background, then you can fast-forward
through these parts, but I find such valuable truths in the
pages of the Bible, truths that help me in my everyday life.
For instance, if you back away enough to look at the whole of
Philippians 4, you will discover that Paul may have revealed
the big secret he was talking about when he wrote the words,
"I have learned the secret of being content in any and every
situation." I think the clues are found in the verses
immediately prior, when Paul is giving instructions to the
Philippians who were facing their own difficulties. I'd like to
focus on just the three big ideas.

First, Paul writes, "Rejoice in the Lord always. I will say it again: Rejoice!" (Philippians 4:4). Do you find yourself asking why he felt he had to say it twice? My editor hates it when I do that. She hates it. I think Paul repeated it because he knew that this behavior seemed totally out of place considering the outward circumstances that he and his readers were suffering. Emotionally, they may have all felt more like giving up, lashing out, or complaining at the top of their lungs. But instead Paul suggests that they rejoice. *You've got to be kidding me*, they must have thought, so he replied, "No, I will say it again: Rejoice!"

The truth is there are moments and settings in which none of us feel like being joyful or happy, and the Bible does acknowledge that there are times to weep and mourn—more words from Solomon the Wise. But in the overarching story of our lives, we can choose to rejoice more than we weep and to celebrate more than we complain. We look beyond what we feel to the bigger picture: we are still alive, shuffling strong, and can count way more good things than bad in our lives. Have I mentioned my grandson, yet?

Next, Paul teaches: "Do not be anxious about anything, but in every situation, by prayer and petition, with thanksgiving, present your requests to God. And the peace of God, which transcends all understanding, will guard your hearts and your minds in Christ Jesus" (Philippians 4:6-7). Notice with this one he ties a kind of pledge from God on the end of the instruction; that is, part of the answer to our prayer will be that the peace of God will guard our hearts and our minds. Wait, isn't that what Solomon said from the beginning? That we need to guard our hearts?

Prayer helps me do that. I'm just speaking from personal experience here. I know some people think religion in general and activities like prayer in particular are just a crutch. Well, I can tell you that it's not a crutch for me. It's more like a walker—a balance-enhancing, weight-bearing, movement-enabling apparatus that serves as a stabilizing force in my life. I don't see the downside to admitting that we might need something that helps us keep moving forward and brings a sense of peace and calm to our hearts and minds.

For me, prayer is the one conversation in which I can be completely honest and vulnerable. I can be the authentic me because I'm speaking to someone who already knows my words before I speak them, my thoughts before I think them, my needs before I present them, and my doubts before I even know that they're there. Being anything less than completely honest when we pray is futile because God already knows everything before we even start. I can say whatever I want to say to God, and he's not surprised or shocked or thinking to himself, *Now, where did all that anger come from?* Of course, if the only thing that comes to mind when you hear the word *prayer* is the pious and polite prayers of some ornate cathedral, then I would say as politely as I can that you don't know prayer, at least my version of it. Nor, dare I say, the biblical version of it.

I love to read the musings of Philip Yancey. His titles alone grab your attention from the very start: *Where Is God When It Hurts?*, *Disappointment With God*, *Church: Why Bother?*, and *What Good Is God?* He kind of tells it like it is, as you might be able to guess. One of my favorite books of his is called *Prayer: Does It Make Any Difference?* This is how he describes authentic prayer: "Prayer allows a place for me to bring my doubts and complaints—in sum, my ignorance—and subject them to the blinding light of a reality I cannot comprehend but can haltingly learn to trust. Prayer is personal, and my doubts take on a different cast as I get to know the Person to whom I bring them." That's what I believe prayer is all about: I'm getting to know God and realizing in every encounter with him that he already knows me—he's just waiting for me to become aware of that fact, because he knows that once I do, I will only pray genuine prayers. Anything less would be meaningless ritual.

It's likely that Paul would agree. He says to take every situation to God in prayer—the ones we like and the ones we don't like, the ones we understand and the ones we don't understand, the ones that seem fair and the ones that seem jarringly unfair. Notice we are to do that with thanksgiving, which takes us back to the *rejoice* idea, and the resulting benefit is that God guards your heart and mind with his peace.

Guards them from what? He guards you from anxiety, because you've just expressed your worries to God; from bitterness, because you've already vented your anger to God; from despair, because in the very act of praying you have shown that there is hope in your heart—hope that God will hear and respond to your prayer.

So, Paul instructs us to be happy and not to worry. Too bad he didn't reverse the order. He might have had a hit song on his hands. Then, Paul gives one last directive: "Finally, brothers and sisters, whatever is true, whatever is noble, whatever is right, whatever is pure, whatever is lovely, whatever is admirable—if anything is excellent or praiseworthy—think about such things" (Philippians 4:8). Again, Paul takes us back to where we started. One of the ways we choose from our hearts to stay upbeat and optimistic is that we refuse to dwell on the negative and we learn to focus on the positive. We think about the right things. We concentrate on what we can still do and not on what we cannot do. It's a heart thing.

About six months after I was diagnosed with Parkinson's, my brother-in-law, Scott, was diagnosed with colon cancer. It was devastating news for our whole family. He had surgery to remove a cancerous tumor that had been blocking his colon and causing excruciating pain—along with ten to twelve inches of his intestines and about twenty lymph nodes from that same area. And to make sure they got everything, the surgery was followed with twelve rounds of chemotherapy over a span of six months. It was an endurance test of his physical, emotional, and spiritual stamina.

Scott wrote about that time:

I learned that I didn't have a lot of control over my

circumstances. All I had the power to do was control my attitude and response to the situation. Sure, I could spend time focusing on what went wrong. I'm in my early 40s. This is a disease that normally strikes people in their sixties, seventies, or eighties. And it is more likely to happen to those who don't take care of their bodies, are heavy drinkers, smokers, overweight, or don't exercise. But none of that was me. Life had thrown me a curve ball, plain and simple. But I made a decision. I would maintain a positive attitude and response and push myself to levels that I didn't think I could complete. I would try to focus on others and inspire and encourage them. I would show everyone the truth of Ralph Waldo Emerson's words: "What lies behind us and what lies before us are tiny matters compared to what lies within us."

So, what did Scott do to prove what lay within him? He did what any cancer surgery and chemo treatment patient would do. In the *middle* of his treatments, he entered a sprint triathlon. Like you would do, right? He had his doctor's permission, but "not my mom's," he admitted. And when we pushed him on the reason he was running, he explained, "Because it's something I've never done before."

Here's what happened. The one triathlon turned out to be only the beginning. He later ran in three 5K races, even as his body weakened during the final rounds of chemo. Because he inspired his doctors, nurses, and everyone else in the community who heard the story, he began to be invited to speak in schools and churches about overcoming adversity and keeping positive despite the difficult circumstances of life. That whole year was very inspirational for all of us who watched Scott run. The happy ending of the story is that he's still running and he's cancer free. Scott did what we all have the power to do. It's what Paul challenged us to do. Don't worry. Be happy. Think on the right things.

We visited Scott and Melanie a few times during that

year of chemo. On one particular morning, I got up early to walk as I usually do. Scott came bounding down the stairs and asked to tag along. How does a triathlon runner "tag along" with a shuffling fool? Well, we did find a way. I stayed close to the sidewalk and, as needed, used that curb trick I'd learned. Scott ran circles around me. Literally. That was the only way to stay close enough to talk. I'm pretty sure we looked ridiculous. When we got back home, we made breakfast for all the sleepyheads still in bed. We can't all be super athletes.

HUMOR

A cheerful heart is good medicine, but a crushed spirit dries up the bones.
—Proverbs 17:22

    I grew up in the southern tip of the state of Alabama, the part of the state my friends and I affectionately referred to as "L.A." (Lower Alabama) in a feeble attempt to sound cooler than any of us would ever be. But once we opened our mouths, the southern drawl removed any possibility that we might have been California-born and bred. That and the red-clay-covered tires on our vehicles. And the smell of the paper mills that drifted across the bay.

    I'll never forget the first time I brought Cheryl home to meet the parents, she blurted out, "What's that horrible, horrible odor?"

    "Home," I replied, a little wounded. I guess it was an acquired aroma. She never acquired it, by the way.

    Yet, Alabama, for all of its renowned backwardness and historical reluctance to accept newfangled ideas—like civil rights, for instance—is really a breathtakingly picturesque place to live. You've got the spectacular foothills in the northernmost part, which mark the beginning of the Appalachian Mountains. You've got the blinding-white, sandy coasts that border the Gulf of Mexico in the south, which I still consider to be some of the most gorgeous beaches in the world. Then, flowing right through the middle of it all, there's the unstoppable Crimson Tide. Well, except for that one forever-in-the-ESPN-highlight-reel return of the missed field goal with no time left on the clock that won the game for Auburn in a recent Iron Bowl. But no one's bitter. There's no animosity. Hey, one of my childhood friends who went to school with me from kindergarten through twelfth grade is now a professor at Auburn, so, I say, "Congratulations! Enjoy the win … until next time. Then Roll Tide again!" But despite the heated football rivalry, the state of Alabama was and is an absolutely *sweet* place to call home. Somebody should probably write a song about the place.

One of my favorite childhood memories of Alabama was the youth camp that we attended every year. It was paradise for a twelve-year-old—a week of sleeping in cabins, hiking in the woods, and swimming in the pool. There were loads of fun activities throughout the day, and an inspirational, come-to-Jesus-style speaker preached every night. Now, four decades later, I have to admit that I don't remember very many of those camp sermons. I was usually too busy thinking about what was going on the next day and which cute girl I should invite to the Friday night banquet—if I ever got up the nerve. The fact of the matter is, out of all the high-energy messages that I fidgeted through during those years and years of listening, only one is forever etched in my memory.

The speaker was Dave Roever, a Vietnam vet who had a remarkable story to share. He had been a riverboat gunner in the Navy, part of the Brown Water Black Berets. Dave was less than a year into his tour when a phosphorus grenade went off in his hand while he prepared to hurl it toward an enemy bunker. The grenade had been struck by a sniper's bullet and exploded six inches from the side of his head. His whole upper body burst into flames and continued to burn as he fell into the water. Most of the right side of his face was burned away down to the skull, and a gaping hole was blown into his chest. He was left blind in his right eye and deaf in his right ear. The medics who airlifted him out thought he was as good as dead, yet miraculously he survived.

That evening at camp, Dave spoke to an absolutely captivated group of campers. We could barely breathe as we looked up at the scarred face and hands of this walking, talking miracle. No one fidgeted that night, I can assure you. We were riveted to our seats. It's easy to understand why this one message stuck.

There's another reason, however, that Dave Roever's story made such an impression on me when he had all of us gathered in the chapel on that warm summer night. He was hilarious. As he told his horrifying tale, there were actually moments we roared with laughter. I remember thinking to myself, *How could anyone go through such terrible pain and suffering and still be able to laugh?* But that's exactly what he did, and his humor was contagious.

I can still vividly recall two details he shared. The first was the nickname he gave himself in the burn unit at the Brooke Army Medical Center in San Antonio, Texas, when he returned to the States. He told everyone that he wanted to be called "Well Done." Why? Because he just felt strongly that one day when he stood before God, there was no way that the Lord could say anything to him but that phrase: "Well done, my good and faithful servant."

Not rare, not medium-well, but well-done! And we laughed because he laughed, maybe nervously at first, but by the end of the night he had put everyone at ease. We were talking about burning flesh and disfigured faces and excruciating pain ... and laughing.

Later in his message came the second memorable detail. He described what happened when his wife saw him for the first time, after his transfer to the Texas facility. In the days before this visit, he witnessed the nightmare that many of his fellow burn ward victims were living. A wife would walk hesitantly up to her husband's bed, take one look at the mutilated body and face, and then quietly slip off her wedding ring and place it on the table next to the bunk. So when

Dave's wife, Brenda, was granted permission to visit, Dave expected the worst.

Unable to recognize him, Brenda actually had to read the name on the chart beside his bed to be sure that it was her husband. Then, she simply bent down to kiss his scarred face and said, "I love you, Dave. Welcome home."

With a whisper, he apologized to her: "I'm so sorry that I won't be good-looking, anymore."

And she immediately answered, "That's OK, Dave. You never were that good-looking in the first place."

As a preteen, I distinctly remember thinking, *I don't know if I could do what she did or face what he faced with that kind of humor and grace.* But I also remember believing that it was exactly what they both needed. The laughter, the witty remarks, the quick comebacks, the twinkle in their eyes as they spoke to one another—all of that was the very thing that enabled them to overcome the sadness and focus on the good. Dave was miraculously alive, they still loved each other dearly, and their story would inspire others to face the future with the same kind of optimism and hope.

OK, maybe I didn't come up with all of that back then. I was only twelve, and there was still that Friday night banquet to worry about. But their example has certainly come back to my mind many times since that night in Alabama, and especially lately. Dave and Brenda chose to laugh when most people expected them to cry. I have decided to do the same.

~

From the very beginning of my own struggle with Parkinson's, I've let the world know that I am going to face this with a large dose of honesty and an even larger dose of humor. I believe the latter helps us swallow the former. So, I laugh.

I laugh for my own sake and for the sake of my family and friends, to put them at ease from the start and to let them know they don't have to avoid any subjects around me. In the spirit of Dave Roever, my wife and I wanted to come up with a nickname right away. She thought my "shuffling fool" moniker was too harsh, so we came up with "Shuffleupagus"—a tribute to a beloved character from our Sesame Street-watching days with our daughters and someone whose belabored movement and slow talk now seems warmly familiar. (No offense, Snuffleupagus.) The name stuck, as you can imagine, and every time we use it, it disarms people and they smile even if they don't think they should.

When my mother-in-law first heard Cheryl call me by that name, she was visibly angry that her daughter could be so insensitive, even if I was just a son-in-law. But then we explained that this was how we wanted to handle my condition—not with quiet whispers behind closed doors, but openly, freely, and ... hilariously. It would be our way of saying that this thing hasn't beaten me and I intend to keep on living and enjoying life.

One of my favorite inspirational posters of all time is of a marsh with a large, white heron looming in the foreground, attempting to swallow a tasty, green frog. The frog's head has already disappeared inside the mouth of the bird, but the frog is squeezing the heron's throat so tightly with his two front feet that it is impossible for him to be swallowed. And the caption reads: "Never, ever give up." That's the message we want to send to everyone we meet.

And we have found that humor is contagious. Our daughters were quick studies. When they first heard that the diagnosis was not just Parkinson's but *young* onset Parkinson's, their immediate reaction was, "Young? The doctor said *young*? What did you do, phone in?" Maybe now they were catching on too well.

My colleagues at work caught on rapidly, too. Recently, our school was hosting a "Dig Pink" volleyball tournament to help raise awareness for breast cancer. The night was a big success. Then a fellow teacher came up and suggested that we host another tournament in the spring, this time for

Parkinson's Disease. I thought it was a great idea.

"What kind of event would we host?" I inquired, a little slow on the uptake.

"Only one option," he replied. "A shuffleboard tournament." I was only upset that he beat me to the punch line.

~

Returning to our old friend Solomon the Wise, the Bible says he spent a lifetime adding to his wisdom. He wrote a thousand and five songs and spoke three thousand proverbs. And although he names a few other contributors, most of the book of Proverbs is attributed to him. Most likely, he penned the one that opened this chapter: "A cheerful heart is good medicine, but a crushed spirit dries up the bones." What I think is amazing about this wise adage is that Solomon seemed to be ahead of his time, medically speaking. For what he simply observed in his day and recorded for posterity has actually been proven to be sound medical advice: a cheerful heart *is* good medicine.

Even though researchers might not all agree on which health benefits have been proven conclusively to be linked, the possible side effects that have been associated with humor and laughter include increasing blood flow and circulation in the body, improving blood pressure, reducing stress and anxiety levels, boosting the body's immune system, helping to curtail depression, relaxing the whole body, and diminishing physical pain. In addition to all these, laughter does the obvious as well. It can improve the mood and outlook of the patient, increase the feelings of overall happiness and well-being, and alleviate, at least temporarily, any sense of tension and fear. There are medications for all of the above, but a good sense of humor will produce some of the same results. And you don't have to stand in the line at the pharmacy.

Solomon goes on to say that the opposite is true as well:

"A crushed spirit dries up the bones." Depression is often described as one of the key predictors of poor health. That's probably because depression leads us into a vicious cycle of self-fulfilling prophecies. We believe we're too sick to do anything about it, which saddens us to the point that we don't and then we get worse, which leads us to the renewed sense that we're too sick to even try and the cycle begins again. The end result, Solomon says, is that our bones dry up, which is a not-so-euphemistic way to say that despair can suck the life out of us until we one day die. Solomon repeats this idea several times in the book of Proverbs, perhaps most obviously in Proverbs 18:14: "The human spirit can endure in sickness, but a crushed spirit who can bear?" We humans are fairly resilient, he seems to say, but if we give in to a sense of hopelessness, the result is almost guaranteed to be detrimental to our health.

So, hopelessness or humor? I'm opting for the latter. It's not because I believe a few good belly laughs will cure me. If that were true, I'd be in enrolled in laughter therapy every day and a laughter yoga group every night. And there really are such things for people with Parkinson's. Instead, I just believe that being able to look at the lighter side of things will keep my spirits up, as well as the spirits of everyone around me, and that's important to me. If all those healthy side effects prove to be true as well, even better. The bottom line is that the ability to see the humor in life helps me cope. When I can throw my head back and laugh wholeheartedly, at times even at myself and my circumstances, that enables me to enjoy every day as a gift from God. In my book, that is indeed a good medicine.

~

One of the sad parts of my pastoral duties is that every once in a while I will have to officiate a funeral. Baby dedications and weddings, I don't mind. Funerals are another story. Now, I believe that there is an afterlife and that it has everything to do with Jesus. The Apostle Paul says in 1 Thessalonians 4 that because we have that hope, we don't grieve like others might grieve who have no hope. That just means that the funerals I do usually feel more like celebrations than times of mourning. The sadness that remains is the sense of loss that we feel when someone passes from our lives. You can hope all you want that you will one day see them again, but that doesn't diminish the fact that the person has been taken from us right now. So, what in the world does a funeral have to do with having a sense of humor?

As I was writing this chapter, a friend of mine called and asked if I would speak at his son's funeral service. I've known the family for years so obviously I said yes. The tough part for me was that Peter, the young man, was only twenty-four years old when he died. He had been one of my students back in high school, and he had been through many hard times in his short life.

When he was just three, he began to have heart trouble, and he finally received a heart transplant about a year prior to his death—on Christmas Day of all days. One week later, they had to amputate his leg due to circulation problems. His dad was devastated that day. I was, as well, and I was supposed to be the man of faith who had all the comforting answers. Peter himself cried, his dad told us later, when he heard the news. "But only for about fifteen minutes," he explained. I wouldn't find out about that, however, until the day of the memorial service.

I remember thinking that Peter would be despondent for weeks after losing his leg. I couldn't have been more wrong. When I checked his Facebook page the next day, he had posted a picture of what remained of his leg. It was wrapped in gauze, huge, round, and swollen, about the size of a big, frozen turkey. Under the picture he had typed, "Happy Thanksgiving, everyone!" That was the Peter I had known since he was a young teenager in my class—always upbeat, always smiling, always looking at the bright side. I was just amazed that he was able to maintain that in the middle of all he was going through.

I went to see him a few days later, bearing gifts. They were books, because that's what I do. I'm a teacher. I assume that everyone loves to read like I do. Peter grunted at the first one. Evidently, my assumption was unfounded. But his eyes lit up when he saw the second one. It was a children's book, with plenty of pictures, which he seemed to like a whole lot more, and he laughed out loud when he saw the title on the cover: *Put Your Best Foot Forward.*

"This is perfect," he grinned, and he kept on grinning for the next eleven months or so. I saw that same ear-to-ear smile when he started rehab a few weeks later wearing a Superman T-shirt and walking up and down fourteen flights of stairs. I saw it again in a photo of the day he got his new temporary leg, this time with a T-shirt that read, "It's all good in the hood." I saw it when he attended the birthday party of a family friend whose little girl was turning four and asked for a "Princesses and Pirates" party theme. Peter came dressed as a pirate with one leg, disguising his prosthetic as a wooden stub. The pictures of him dancing around with the birthday girl were priceless.

He died two months later, and more than five hundred people attended the standing-room-only memorial service to pay tribute to his life. In the eulogies, he was described as an inspiration to others, someone with the ability to light up a room with his smile, his energy, and his undying sense of humor. He was commended for always being strong and upbeat, although he had more reasons than most to be the total opposite type of person. In the end, he died of physical problems he could not overcome, but as I said at the funeral, ultimately he won because he never let the obstacles that he faced keep him from enjoying life to the fullest and spurring on others to do the same. (Here's to you, Peter!)

~

When we moved from Costa Rica to Honduras, Cheryl and I graduated from the Spanish Language Institute with flying colors. We were considered near-fluent speakers when we got on the plane and took the short flight to Honduras. However, when we disembarked and stepped into the hot, muggy airport of San Pedro Sula, we noticed right away that we could barely understand a word that anyone said to us.

What we hadn't realized was that spoken Spanish varies between regions of Latin America as much as English does throughout the United States and the world. Imagine a good old boy from Georgia conversing with a native Bostonian for the first time or a Texan talking with a Londoner. You'd almost need subtitles. It took us weeks, if not months, to make the adjustment in our hearing and speaking skills before we were communicating successfully once more. The funny part was that when we returned to Costa Rica a year later for a visit, our former teachers observed that we had picked up a Honduran accent, and they did not approve.

But I discovered something in the process of learning a new language, bad accent or no. If I was willing to make linguistic mistakes publicly and then laugh at myself when I figured out what I had actually said, that self-deprecating sense of humor won the hearts of the people I worked with. Better yet, it helped me to master the language even more quickly because my Spanish-speaking friends felt at liberty to point out my errors without worrying about offending me. A sense of humor was the key.

The opposite was also true. If language learners showed resentment when corrected, the people who could have served as the best teachers in the world instead shut down and let the offended fend for themselves. Almost every time, the end result was a botched learning opportunity. One co-worker I served with for a few years never really mastered the Spanish language because he displayed precisely this attitude. Even in his farewell speech, he blundered badly.

He was trying to explain that his past could be divided into two separate parts: the life lived before he met God and the time since. It was a heart-warming testimonial, but he made one, tiny error. Instead of using the correct Spanish words for "my past," he used another word meaning "my rear end." When the Honduran guests that evening heard him mistakenly say that the latter was divided into two parts, there were shouts of agreement and laughter from all around the room. It was a natural reaction.

If my friend had only been able to laugh at himself in that moment, he would have endeared himself forever to the men and women who gathered to honor him that night. They would have given him a standing ovation. Instead, he left annoyed and a little insulted. Everyone there felt badly.

I took a very different approach. In every scenario, in every relationship, in every group setting, I asked that everyone become my teacher and correct me on every misspoken word, especially the funny ones. My Honduran colleagues did so reluctantly at first but gradually learned that they could do so freely with me. They would laugh themselves to tears at times, and then, when they finally caught their breath, they would let me in on the joke. I usually laughed harder than they did. I made as many mistakes as the next guy, maybe more, but the laughter eased the tension on every occasion.

My wife did the same. Once, when we had distinguished guests in our home for a meal, Cheryl announced to everyone that the food was ready and that we could now pray over the meal. At least, that is what she meant to say. That night she used the word *llorar* (cry) instead of *orar* (pray), and all the guests in that moment simultaneously began to weep loudly. It took us a minute but then we caught it, too, and we laughed until we cried. It was an evening we would talk about for years.

Many of the mistakes I made cannot be repeated in this G-rated book, but I had a few that would pass the censors. At a large church of several hundred people, I once preached a whole sermon on Jesus being the Good Shepherd. I just had him watching over bees (*avejas*) instead of sheep (*ovejas*). I knew I had heard several people giggling but didn't put two and two together until I was nearly done and finally yelled, "What?" The entire congregation began to make buzzing sounds like a bee. My reputation had preceded me, it seemed. I defiantly said that Jesus made a pretty good beekeeper, as well, and they roared.

My biggest teaching moment came when I interpreted for a guest speaker at the annual conference for all the pastors of our particular denomination, with probably close to a thousand ministers and their spouses in attendance.

My main job in Honduras was teaching in the Bible schools, and my two favorite classes to teach were about how to interpret and to preach the Bible—hermeneutics and homiletics, respectively. All over the country, I taught classes large and small. In every one of those classrooms, the students became the teachers for me, as well, and we shared hilarious moments together.

So, in that conference, hundreds of those in attendance were my former students. As the English-speaking guest was at the height of his message, he delivered the line, "And Paul was thrown in the dungeon." I promptly translated the phrase, and the whole crowd broke into spatterings of laughter. The speaker stopped midsentence and repeated the line, and I did, too, at which point everyone really got tickled. Then it seemed like a thousand voices yelled out the correct word. Apparently, I had sentenced Paul to hard time in a pumpkin (*calabaza*) instead of a dungeon (*calabozo*). I told them that I was just making sure they were listening.

We spent eleven entertaining years in Honduras and made many dear friends. I'd like to think we were known for our deep spirituality, hard work, and dedication to the cause, but often when I met my former students and we had the opportunity to catch up, they would recall something funny I had said. And they thanked me for being vulnerable with them. Some even wept when we left, and it wasn't because we used the wrong word this time. I think it was because we had opened ourselves up to people and taught them that it was

OK to laugh, to enjoy life, and to serve others with a joy in our hearts. Good old Solomon said it best in Ecclesiastes 3:12: "I know that there is nothing better for people than to be happy and to do good while they live."

~

    An old adage says, "Laugh, and the world laughs with you; weep, and you weep alone." Actually, it's the first line to the poem "Solitude," by Ella Wheeler Wilcox, originally published in 1883. Its essential message is that happy people attract others, while unhappy people drive them away. The idea is repeated throughout the poem in lines such as: "Rejoice, and men will seek you; grieve, and they turn and go," and "Be glad, and your friends are many; be sad, and you lose them all." It's the difference between doing life with others and doing it alone. Laughter, at least according to Wilcox, is one of the deciding factors.

    We're naturally drawn toward folks who seem to always have a good time, who make us laugh, and who are fun to be around. You know the feeling. You're at a dinner party and one group seems like it's full of people having the best time there. You secretly want to switch seats with someone at that table. We like to hang around those kinds of people because we walk away with a slight spring in our step. We actually feel better about ourselves. Why is that?

    One reason is because, for a few moments, we allow ourselves to forget about our problems and concerns. Our load feels suddenly lighter. But I think the main reason is because we let our guard down when we laugh. Our bodies and minds relax, and we let ourselves lose control for a moment. Let's face it. Laughing is a vulnerable activity. When we really do it right, our mouths are typically wide-open, tears may be rolling down our cheeks, and strange noises come from somewhere deep inside of us.

    Think about all the different ways people can laugh. There are gigglers, wheezers, squealers, chucklers, snorters, guffawers, snickerers, cacklers, howlers, weepers, even chortlers—although I can't say that I've ever chortled, personally. How would I know? Does anyone really know what *chortling* means?

And if you add motions, there are clappers, rib-grabbers, pointers, back-patters, head-back-throwers, mouth-coverers, shoulder-shakers, knee-slappers, and knuckle-knockers. That last one is my personal favorite because it's a mannerism my wife practices when she really gets tickled. She knocks on the table, knocks on the dash, knocks on the counter—basically, on whatever is close by. I'm not kidding. Just ask my daughters. In fact, ask them to mimic her. They love to do that for a crowd.

The way we laugh is unique to each one of us and at times can be a little embarrassing. So, when we are willing to let our true selves be seen in the form of laughter, what we are really doing is letting go of our ego and pride. And in doing so, we are emboldened to let other things go as well, including our tension, our stress, our inhibitions, and even the social masks we wear and the public personas we try to maintain. No wonder the load feels lighter when we laugh. It's like a therapy session for the soul. It's like a really good medicine. Someone should probably write that down for future generations.

Not too long ago, my Parkinson's buddy, Vince, went into the hospital for back surgery. As I often do in my role as a pastor, I went early that morning to pray with him before the surgery. My intention was to do so quickly and get out of the way. However, they had him wearing what looked like control-top panty hose and before we knew it, Vince, his wife, and I were chortling up a storm, joking about any and everything. When I looked down at my phone and realized how much time had passed, I apologized for doing a stand-up comedy routine instead of saying a prayer.

"Actually," Vince countered, "the laughter was exactly what I needed." He did let me pray with him, too, but I knew what he meant.

A day spent in laughter with the ones you love and cherish is one of the most significant bonding times you can have. On quite a few occasions, my girls have brought me to the point of such uncontrollable, red-faced, impossible-to-catch-my-breath episodes of laughter that I have actually had to beg them to stop for a minute so I wouldn't implode. I guess we can add that to the list of laughers: beggars-for-breath. I wouldn't trade those moments for anything in the world.

HOPE

Anyone who is among the living has hope—even a live dog is better off than a dead lion! —Ecclesiastes 9:4

Solomon always had a way with words. He's credited for three books of the Bible: Proverbs, Song of Songs, and Ecclesiastes. Ecclesiastes happens to be one of my favorites in a weird sort of way, mainly because it's so real—a little pessimistic, but real. There are scholars who try to paint the book as ultimately about enjoying life as a gift from God, but Solomon doesn't really get there until the twelfth and final chapter. Up until then, his favorite word is *meaningless*. His opening line is revealing and sets the tone for the entire book. "'Meaningless! Meaningless!' says the Teacher. 'Utterly meaningless! Everything is meaningless'" (Ecclesiastes 1:2).

And just in case there's any doubt about what Solomon means by *everything*, he spells it out over the next eleven and a half chapters. Study, pleasures, wisdom, and foolishness are all meaningless. So are work, toil, achievement, advancement, dreaming, wealth, laughter, youth, and vigor. Essentially, he says everything in life now and to come is meaningless. He does say that we should enjoy life, but read the whole line in which that phrase is found to get the context: "Enjoy life

with your wife, whom you love, all the days of
this meaningless life that God has given you under the sun—
all your meaningless days. For this is your lot in life and in
your toilsome labor under the sun" (Ecclesiastes 9:9). He was
quite the motivational speaker.

The king does finally get to a more spiritual-sounding
answer in the final verses of the last chapter, in which he
writes his summation of his search for meaning. Here's his
conclusion: "Fear God and keep his commandments, for this
is the duty of all mankind" (Ecclesiastes 12:13). This is
something you would expect from someone writing in the
Bible, right? But that's not before he takes one more parting
shot in the verses immediately prior to our text:
"'Meaningless!' says the Teacher. 'Everything is
meaningless!'" (Ecclesiastes 12:8).

But right in the middle of all of that less-than-
encouraging talk, he plants this one little seed of optimism.
"Anyone who is among the living has hope—even a live dog
is better off than a dead lion!" (Ecclesiastes 9:4). Well, I didn't
say it was gushing with optimism, but it's there. In this
chapter, Solomon is talking about the common destiny
awaiting us all—the righteous and the wicked, the good and
the bad, the pure and the impure, those who worship God
and those who do not—and that destiny is that we will all die.
Once that happens, there's no further possibility of knowing
more, loving more, or taking part in anything more under the
sun. But as long as we are still alive on the planet, there's
hope—hope to change, hope to learn, hope to be rewarded,
hope to live and love and laugh, hope to become wiser with
every passing day. That's where we started, if you remember,
with that simple prayer: "Teach us to number our days, that
we may gain a heart of wisdom." You can only do that if
you're alive and kicking.

Basically, as long as we still have breath, we have hope.
Alexander Pope wrote: "Hope springs eternal in the human
breast." It's built into us, whether you believe that's by God's
design or evolutionary necessity. The fact remains that the

human heart always seems to want the best possible outcome, the happy-ever-after ending. We look for that to happen, but even when it doesn't, we tend to wake up the next day hoping again that it will. There's a great line from the book of Lamentations, in which Jeremiah writes in the midst of his affliction and bitterness of soul: "Yet this I call to mind and therefore I have hope: Because of the Lord's great love we are not consumed, for his compassions never fail. They are new every morning; great is your faithfulness" (Lamentations 3:21-23). Jeremiah's hope is directly tied to the renewable resources of God's love, compassion, and faithfulness, but the part I want to emphasize is that it's new every morning. As long as we still have breath, we have hope.

~

Earlier, I introduced you to my brother-in-law, Scott. He's the one who ran a sprint triathlon or two during the months he was going through his chemotherapy. He also decided to chronicle his treatments each week since he would be stuck in the chair hooked up to an IV for hours at a time, anyway. In the beginning, he just planned to send an update to about ten people to share his thoughts and struggles and to express his determination to overcome what he referred to as the most difficult path of his life. Yet, what started as a small, encouraging email dubbed, "Thoughts from the Chemo Chair," grew to include hundreds of people, including the senior executives of the multinational company for which he worked. He talked about courage and endurance and having the right attitude along the way. The top brass of his company would later honor him with their Presidential Award. He was one of four chosen out of a total of eight hundred employees as part of their Circle of Excellence program—not just for what he endured, but how he had inspired all of them in the process and changed the culture of the entire company. His wife, Melanie, likes to brag that he was the only one that night who received a standing ovation.

And I think my sister has every right to be proud of her man.

What I found especially intriguing was his last post of the series, on the twelfth and final week. Listen to what he wrote:

> I've come to the end of my chemo sessions. After the first couple of sessions, I wondered how I could make it through twelve. I found my answer as I tried to focus on inspiring and encouraging others. Life is about making choices. How we choose to react or respond to the circumstances and obstacles placed in our lives is what defines us. Above all, there is hope. I have hope. I have hope in someone much bigger than I am. I have hope for an eventual cure for cancer. I have hope for tomorrow.

But what does it mean to have hope? To hope is to eagerly desire something to become real or to be true. We use the word almost every day of our lives, almost like a wish. I *hope* you have a fun-filled birthday. I *hope* they have a safe trip home. I *hope* our team makes the playoffs. I *hope* I pass the exam. I *hope* my insurance company covers all the expenses. That last one is what we might refer to as hoping against hope, a rather odd turn of phrase, don't you think? It means to hope for something when there is no hope.

The point is that we all have things for which we hope. We hope for big things—*I really hope we win that Powerball lottery*; and small—*I hope the traffic light stays green a few seconds longer.* We hope for good things—*I hope you get to sign on the house you wanted*; and bad—*I hope the blue bird-of-paradise flies up your nose.* We can also hope for significant things—*I hope they find a cure for cancer and Parkinson's and AIDS*; or insignificant ones—*I hope this shirt makes my eyes pop* and *makes me look twenty pounds thinner.* That's another example of hoping against hope. But no matter what they are, we all have hopes.

Some people, though, think of hope as mere wishful thinking, some kind of mental trick that we use to help us escape from reality, or worse. Nietzsche wrote that hope is "the worst of all evils for it prolongs the torments of man." I wholeheartedly disagree. Hope is what gives us the will to go on, to fight another day, to keep on trying, and never give up. It's not running from reality, it's staring it down with determination and maybe some good old-fashioned grit—the toughness of character we all need when trials interrupt our lives.

The image that comes to my mind is the ruddy-faced shepherd boy David, of Bible fame, running toward the hulking champion Goliath, instead of away from him. There was seemingly no chance of David winning, and yet he succeeded because he had a tenacity that was equal parts perseverance, courage, and hope. Well, that, and he was a crackerjack shot with a sling. The perseverance part just meant that David had been through tough battles before. That's what the word *perseverance* literally means, through severity. To be specific, David explains that while tending his father's flocks, he had rescued stolen sheep from both the mouth of a lion and a bear. And, apparently, not just from a distance, either. He claims that he chased the animal down, struck it, and then rescued the sheep from its mouth. And when it turned on him, he seized it by its hair and killed it. Me? I would have just crossed those two sheep off my inventory. I have a hard time picturing myself running after a lion.

There was no doubt about his courage, then. His intelligence, maybe, but not his courage. We see his courage when he arrives on the scene in 1 Samuel 17. The undefeated Goliath had taunted the armies of Israel for forty days and all of the so-called seasoned warriors of the Israeli army fled from the mere sight of him, dismayed and terrified. Then David shows up to bring his brothers food from home, hears the taunts, and immediately volunteers to fight him. Evidently, David's past victories had emboldened him and made him fearless. He tells King Saul that he'll do the job, and Saul offers him his own coat of armor, helmet, and sword. Ultimately, that all proves to be too big for David, so he goes in with just his sling and five stones.

We all know what happens next. It's one of the most famous stories in the world. We use the David and Goliath metaphor for almost every underdog scenario we talk about—in sports, in politics, in business, in war, in everything.

So, that's perseverance and courage. But where and how does hope come into the picture? The first thing you have to realize is that *hope* in the biblical sense is not just blindly yearning for something to be true. It's more substantive than that. It's way more than mere wishful thinking and believing that if we somehow wish hard enough, what we wished for will come true. No, in the Bible, hope has more to do with a sense of confidence or trust based on what has already happened, which in turn gives us the faith and hope to face the future. David faced Goliath with this hope in his heart: "The Lord who rescued me from the paw of the lion and the paw of the bear will rescue me from the hand of this Philistine" (1 Samuel 17:37). David is saying, "God's done it before, and he can do it again."

You find this kind of hope all through the Scriptures— again, not the wishful thinking, throw-the-coin-in-the- fountain kind, but more of a quiet, trusting, confident hope. The writer of Hebrews describes hope as a firm and secure anchor (6:19). He defines faith as confidence in what we hope for and assurance about what we do not see (11:1) and then he lists a whole chapter of people who lived that way. He admonishes his readers to hold unswervingly to the hope they had professed and then he tells them why: "For he who promised is faithful" (Hebrews 10:23). As David said earlier in the Old Testament: God's done it before, and he can do it again.

Speaking of David, years after his encounter with Goliath, he would pen these words about hope in Psalm 25: "In you, Lord my God, I put my trust. I trust in you; do not let me be put to shame. ... No one who hopes in you will ever be put to shame. ... Show me your ways, Lord, teach me your paths. Guide me in your truth and teach me, for you are God my Savior, and my hope is in you all day long" (Psalm 25:1-5). Did you notice how the words *hope* and *trust* are used interchangeably? Hope is all about trusting.

So, that's what I'm doing. I'm trusting. That's what I believe Scott meant in his posts. He's trusting in someone bigger than he is. He's trusting that there will be an eventual cure for the disease he had to face. He's trusting that he will get to live another day and keep on fighting. Me, too.

Now, I know that first one—trusting in someone bigger—depends on whether you even believe in God. I do, and that gives me a great deal of peace and comfort. I pray this prayer all the time, both for others and myself:

> God, I'm trusting in your goodness, that you know what's best for me. And I'm trusting in your power, that you have the ability to heal me if you want to. I'll still believe the first one, Lord, even if the second one doesn't take place. But, just for the record, you know which answer I prefer.

That may be a little too presumptuous for some folks, but I don't know how to pray any other way.

There are two passages in the Bible where this kind of prayer is lived out. One is in the Old Testament book of Daniel, where three Hebrew captives are about to be thrown into a furnace for not bowing down to the king's golden idol. The king's name is Nebuchadnezzar, and when he questions the three, they answer him with these words of hope: "If we are thrown into the blazing furnace, the God we serve is able to deliver us from it, and he will deliver us from Your Majesty's hand. But even if he does not, we want you to know, Your Majesty, that we will not serve your gods or worship the image of gold you have set up" (Daniel 3:17-18). They knew that God could, and they believed that he would, but even if he didn't, they would not cease to trust and obey their God. That story ends happily, incidentally, because God does deliver them.

The second passage does not end well, however, and that's ironic considering who is praying. It's Jesus, the night before he would be crucified, the night he was betrayed. The Scriptures say that he prayed this prayer so hard that he sweated drops of blood. He admitted to his disciples that his soul was overwhelmed with sorrow to the point of death. Realizing what was about to happen to him over the next twenty-four hours, Jesus spoke pretty honestly to God: "Father, if you are willing, take this cup from me" (Luke 22:42). The cup he refers to is the agony he would go through the rest of that night and all the next day. So, Jesus is actually praying that he might be spared from that suffering. That didn't happen, which is good news for all of us, but it wasn't so great for Jesus.

Now, here's where the hope and trust come in. You can hear it in the second half of his prayer: "Yet not my will, but yours be done" (Luke 22:42). He trusted his life and circumstances, his body and soul, to the one who had sent him. His prayer is fairly straightforward: "I'd prefer this answer, but I trust you if it's the other." That's become the model for my prayers over the last few years. I hope that God will heal me. I trust him even if he doesn't.

I've seen God do both. Cheryl and I firmly believe he healed our daughter of seizure activity in the brain. She had one twelve-minute epileptic seizure when she was five. The pediatric neurologist, after extensive testing, told us that she would have seizures for the rest of her life. We prayed and asked everyone we knew to pray with us, and she hasn't had a single episode since that prognosis. I thought about that fact recently when she graduated from college. We firmly believe God answered our prayers. Through the years, we've witnessed him doing the same for others, as well.

Could it have been just a coincidence with our daughter? Yes. Could it have been a misdiagnosis? Maybe, but it's not likely. Could there have been multiple natural explanations? Perhaps. But we believe God granted us a small miracle, and we are forever grateful to him. And yet, truth be told, we've also seen times when God didn't answer—many times, in fact. But that doesn't stop us from believing that he can and hoping that he will. That's the quiet, sure, and confident hope we have in him.

~

This next part may sound strange, especially after all the Bible references and religious jargon I've used in the previous pages, but it's true nonetheless. I also have great faith and hope in science. I know that in our culture many people view faith and science as archenemies and believe that the two concepts should not even be used in the same sentence. You have to choose sides, they say. You're either for the naturalistic explanation of the universe or the supernatural one, but you can't have both.

Why not? I believe that both science and God's revelation of himself are valuable but limited sources of truth. I'm rooting for science to solve more and more of the world's mysteries, including, but not restricted to, a viable cure for Parkinson's. I want more science, not less. I just think that science unnecessarily precludes even the possibility of a supernatural explanation before it even starts. Why not just follow where the evidence leads, even if that opens the door to the likelihood that something beyond the natural might indeed exist? Something like God?

But I also believe that God's revelation of himself is limited. It would seem at times that he purposely obscures himself when he should be blatantly obvious. Now, don't get me wrong. I believe that God has revealed enough about himself through the Scriptures so that we can have a relationship with him, as strange as that may sound to some. But I don't think the Bible even comes close to revealing everything there is to know about God. In fact, the second that God fits into our theological mold, he ceases to be God and becomes instead a construct of our own making. That's why I tell my students all the time that I am at least partially agnostic. I believe we can know God but not fully nor completely. I believe all theologians should be a great deal more humble about their theology.

All that to say this: I have great hope in science and the medical research that is being done all around the world. I think I would even say I'm using that word *hope* in the biblical sense of the word, that is, a sense of confidence or trust based on what has already happened, which in turn gives me the faith and hope to face the future. Medical breakthroughs have changed so much about our lives. They have eradicated some diseases and greatly enhanced the treatment of others. I'm confident that we will one day find a cure for cancer and Parkinson's and Alzheimer's and everything else that seems right now to be unbeatable.

As I write these words, there is talk of a better levodopa on the horizon that would more consistently maintain therapeutic levels of the medication in the body. If that proves to be true, then patients with Parkinson's could actually see fewer symptoms for longer periods of time. Go science!

At the "Living Well with Parkinson's Disease" symposium that I mentioned earlier, the first session of the day was an update on Parkinson's therapies and research. The presenter spoke of new delivery methods, such as a pump straight to the small intestine and an inhaler straight to the lungs, both of which would get the medicine more quickly and evenly into the bloodstream, which is a good thing. There was also excitement about a new PERK inhibitor that aided in the cessation of brain cell death, which is essential in the treatment of neurodegenerative diseases like Alzheimer's and Parkinson's. All of this is beyond my expertise, but what I wanted to point out is that with all of these announcements, do you know what word they kept repeating? *Hope.* Not the wishful thinking kind, mind you, but the extensively-researched, peer-reviewed, clinically proven variety of hope. I'm rooting for all of the above. Go science!

~

So, I have hope—in God, in science, and in tomorrow. Now, I totally get that none of us are guaranteed tomorrow. I'm long past the "I am invincible!" stage of my youth and the thinking that I will never die, or at least past believing that the day is so far off I shouldn't let it even cross my mind. Even the Bible says that we shouldn't boast about what we'll do tomorrow, because our life is like a mist that appears for a little while and then vanishes. That's James talking there. Undoubtedly, he was influenced by Solomon, who probably just forgot to add to his list: "Tomorrow is meaningless, too." Yet, I do have this hope and confidence that I will see tomorrow, primarily because I have this idea stuck in my brain that God might still want to use my life in some way.

~

I'll never forget the summer of 1995. My family and I had returned to the States the previous year for our furlough, a twelve-month working sabbatical spent back "home" after living in Costa Rica and Honduras for four years. We went to visit my parents in Georgia, and, when our first day there dawned with a cloudless, blue sky, my dad and I decided on the spur of the moment to take a canoe trip down the Coosawattee River. We put in near the re-reg dam at Carter's Lake and planned to paddle downstream about ten miles or so. The water level was a little low, typical for the summer, so we did have to haul the canoe over a sandbar or two, but otherwise it was a relaxing way to spend a morning. We talked and paddled as needed but mostly just quietly enjoyed the scenic splendor that surrounded us.

We were a few hours into our journey when we heard what we thought sounded like thunder somewhere far off in the distance—deep, rumbling thunder. We looked up at the clear skies through the opening of the trees above us, saw nothing ominous, and thus continued paddling unhurriedly along. Besides, there was no good place to take out. We were floating through a section of the river with privately owned properties on both sides, with three- to four-foot embankments to our left and right, and barbwire fences running along the tops of the embankments. That was OK, though, because we thought we had plenty of time.

In less than thirty minutes, however, the sun had disappeared behind dark clouds that rolled in with a vengeance, and all of a sudden the bottom dropped out of the sky. The rain came down so hard that it felt like we were sitting under a gutter spout. We started bailing as quickly as possible with anything we could find; yet, even so, the rain was winning.

Then the lightning started, and it felt unusually close. You know how people count between a flash of lightning and the rumble of thunder? However many seconds they reach, that's how many miles away the lightning is, right? We couldn't get past one. We frantically paddled the canoe under the canopy of a nearby tree to try to reduce the amount of water coming in, but there we sat in an aluminum canoe, on the side of a river, in the middle of a fierce lightning storm. I prayed under my breath as intensely as I knew how.

We both did live to tell the story. The storm blew over our particular spot on the river over the course of the next hour and the hair on my head finally laid flat again. We awkwardly clung to the embankment while we tipped the canoe over to empty all the water out and quickly resumed our trip, drenched to the bone. We talked less and paddled more, and we made it to the bridge that marked the spot where we would take out without further incident. The sun came out and the rest of the day was once again gorgeous— soggy, but gorgeous.

We tied the canoe to the top of the truck and started home. I let out a sigh of relief and confessed to Dad that for a few moments there on the river, I was probably as frightened as I had ever been in my life.

"I actually thought we were going to die," I said, perhaps a little overdramatically.

"I wasn't," he said confidently. "I knew we'd be OK."

"Really?" I asked, surprised. "How did you know that?"

"Because I don't believe that God is finished with you, yet." It was a very nice dad-to-son thing to say and, at the same time, humbling to hear. I looked straight ahead and mumbled back that I hadn't been quite so sure about my future in the heat of the moment. For a minute or two back there—or maybe closer to sixty—I thought for sure my number was up. I know, I know. What a man of faith, right?

~

Have you ever asked yourself where that phrase came from? *Your number is up.* Most people would probably say it refers to the practice of clients taking a number when they enter a crowded place of business. When the individual's number is called, then he or she is next to be served. That person is up, we say. For some reason, however, we have come to use the phrase to refer to the time of our death. It's as if the universe or fate or God gives us all a number when we're born and we live until something or someone calls our number. Once those digits are announced, there's no way around it. Your number is up.

The Bible teaches something very similar. And no, this time, it wasn't Solomon who said it. His father, David, did. I've already referenced the verse a couple of times during the course of this book, but allow me to return to it once more, this time with a little more of the context of the surrounding verses:

> You have searched me, Lord, and you know me. You know when I sit and when I rise; you perceive my thoughts from afar. You discern my going out and my lying down; you are familiar with all my ways. Before a word is on my tongue, you, Lord, know it

completely. You hem me in behind and before, and you lay your hand upon me. Such knowledge is too wonderful for me, too lofty for me to attain.

Where can I go from your Spirit? Where can I flee from your presence? If I go up to the heavens, you are there; if I make my bed in the depths, you are there. If I rise on the wings of the dawn, if I settle on the far side of the sea, even there your hand will guide me, your right hand will hold me fast ... .

For you created my inmost being; you knit me together in my mother's womb. I praise you because I am fearfully and wonderfully made; your works are wonderful, I know that full well. My frame was not hidden from you when I was made in the secret place, when I was woven together in the depths of the earth. Your eyes saw my unformed body; all the days ordained for me were written in your book before one of them came to be.

How precious to me are your thoughts, God! How vast is the sum of them! Were I to count them, they would outnumber the grains of sand—when I awake, I am still with you (Psalm 139:1-10, 13-18).

I do believe God gave me a number. In fact, he ordained that number before I was born, conceived, or existed as a twinkle in my dad's eye. I talk to my high school students every year about these verses, and I always ask them the big question: If it were possible, would you want to know that final number? Their answers are usually mixed, and then they always ask how I would answer the question. I say the same thing every time: Definitely not. Ignorance is bliss, I tell them, and I'm all about the bliss, at least in this case. Besides, I think it would really mess me up to know what's going to happen. If I had known at twenty-five that I would have

Parkinson's before I was fifty, what would that have done to my life? Would I have made better choices or worse ones? I have no idea.

But there's a truth in this passage that is even more significant to me. Not only does God know both my beginning and ending dates, he also knows me intimately in all the moments in between. He knows my every movement, my every thought, and my every word before I can speak. There's nowhere in the universe I can go that he's not already there, that he's not with me. And, apparently, he's thinking of me so often, his thoughts are as impossible to count as the sand on the seashore.

When I stop and reflect on the fact that God knows me and walks with me through each and every moment of my life, I'm overwhelmed. I like the way David says it: "Such knowledge is too wonderful for me, too lofty for me to attain." I'm with you, David. Our finite minds are not sufficiently equipped to grasp such complete knowledge and infinite awareness, and on top of it all, unconditional love.

Yet, beyond inspiring a sense of awe, do you know what else the God-knows-me-intimately truth does for me? It helps me trust in whatever ending date he has ordained for me, whether that day happens to be fast approaching or decades away. Anyone who has such perfect knowledge of me, my life and my place in time and history, from beginning to end, can certainly plan my life better than I can. God probably looks at all of us and thinks, *What rookies!*

The God-knows-me-intimately truth also makes me genuinely thankful for every day I'm given and fills me with hope at the prospect of yet another tomorrow. Every morning when I wake up, I whisper this prayer: "Thank you, God, for today and for the gifts of life and breath and health. And thank you for walking with me through each day from start to finish."

That's basically what David said toward the close of this psalm: "When I awake, I am still with you." That's a good feeling—a confidence booster that gives me hope.

And hope keeps me shuffling forward, one tomorrow at a time, using every second wisely, trying not to waste a single day, focusing on the things that really matter. Hey, maybe somewhere along the way I'll gain that heart of wisdom. Maybe I've already started. There's always hope.

ACKNOWLEDGMENTS

Give to everyone what you owe them: If you owe taxes, pay taxes; if revenue, then revenue; if respect, then respect; if honor, then honor.
—Romans 13:7

I don't really need a verse to motivate me to express my gratitude to all the people who have helped me find a way forward. I just liked the way this one sounded.

First of all, to Cheryl: I hope I say this enough. I'm so glad you chose to do life with me. Thanks for sticking with me all these years. You have bewitched me—body and soul—and I love, I love, I love you.

To Brittany, Lauren, and Sarah: From the first moments I laid eyes on each one of you, I was undone. All I have hoped for ever since was not to blow it. You must know, surely you must know, it was all for you.

To my parents, Tommy and Nelda Woodall: For the depth of my roots and the strength of my wings, I am indebted to both of you. We all are.

To Joe: You started all this with a simple text … and I am forever grateful. You lit a fire in me that I cannot seem to put out. I have been, and always shall be, your friend.

To Kristen: Thank you for your wordsmith skills beyond compare. It is your superpower. Well, that and sippy-cup dodging. I would have been lost without you. And to Tim: I'm touched that you read this book. Who knew? Thank you for making it possible for others to do the same.

To Marie and Heather: Thank you for introducing me to all the wonderful people of the Parkinson Association of the Carolinas, none more dedicated than the two of you. You have opened my eyes to a whole new world of opportunities to serve and I'm enjoying every minute.

To Dr. Iyer: Thank you for making an extremely annoying disease a little less annoying for so many people. You and your staff have been a blessing and are a credit to the entire Carolinas Healthcare System. And just for the record, I'm still holding out for that cure.

To God: I'll never get over how you demonstrated your love to each one of us. You sent your one and only Son into the world that we might live through him. Who does that? You do. You did.

NOTES

Page 29
Tolkien, J.R.R., *The Fellowship of the Rings*, volume one of *The Lord of the Rings*. (New York: Ballantine Books, 1965).

Page 38
Lewis, C.S. *The Problem of Pain*. (New York: Macmillan Publishing Company, 1962).

Page 72
"Live Like You Were Dying," words and music by Tim Nichols and Craig Wiseman © by 2004 Warner Tamerlane Music Corp. (BMI) and Big Loud Shirt (ASCAP). Produced by Curb Records.

Pages 75-76
Michael J. Fox on *The Late Show with David Letterman*, aired on CBS, November 12, 2013.

Page 84
"Martha Dandridge Custis Washington," The White House, http://www.whitehouse.gov/about/martha-dandridge-custis-washington.

Page 87
Yancey, Phillip. *Prayer: Does It Make a Difference?* (Grand Rapids, Michigan: Zondervan, 2010).

Pages 92-94
For more about Dave Roever, visit daveroever.org.

Page 103
Wilcox, Ella Wheeler, "Solitude," *Poems of Passion*. (Chicago: Belford, Clarke & Company, 1889, first published in 1883).

CPSIA information can be obtained
at www.ICGtesting.com
Printed in the USA
LVOW10s1514030517
533132LV00008B/630/P